Intermittent Fasting for Women Over 50

The Ultimate Guide with Recipes to Lose Weight, Promote longevity, and Increase Energy with Intermittent Fasting and Autophagy.

By Amy J. Moore

Table of Content

Introduction:

In circles where people strive to find ways to reduce caloric intake without harming their workout goals, intermittent fasting has become very popular and still allows them to lose weight during strength training.

Intermittent fasting, in a nutshell, is a quick and straightforward way to lower your clerical intake so you can achieve your weight loss without hunger plans or other fad diets. It is not only meant to clean up the system, as many people believe. You don't have to worry too much about the types of food you eat while you're not fasting. You are allowing your food choices a sense of freedom.

It relieves the high anxiety that is present when it comes to most diets. Many times, we feel wholly restricted and constrained. Nevertheless, this strategy leaves not only the freedom to choose what we don't like to eat, but also the opportunity to restore balance and equilibrium to our intermittent dead fasting as a lifestyle can bring about lifetime improvements. Start but take it slow at first and really learn to listen to what your body is trying to tell you in the first few weeks. If you feel underfed, change it a bit, your body will say to you, but it will need to go through the same withdrawal at any time, especially at first, and it is essential to learn how to differentiate these signals. You also need to factor in word any workout routine that you might be engaged in on your intermittent fasting plans.

The most important thing about intermittent fasting to remember is that it's not just a diet plan, but also a lifestyle. To get the best possible results from it, you need to be helpful to it. Your fasting should be something you're looking forward to.

The chapters in this book shall deal with intermittent fasting, which helps you to lose weight, promote longevity, increase energy, and more. Also, this diet plan can be easier to follow than other fasting types. People who do intermittent fasting should focus on eating whole foods high in fiber, and they should stay hydrated all day.

Chapter 1: Basic of Intermittent Fasting

Intermittent fasting (IF) is, today, one of the most common fitness and health trends in the world. Consumers use it to lose weight, improve health, and make their lives easier. Many studies demonstrate that it can have powerful effects on your body and brain, and can even help you live longer. This is the ultimate guide to intermittent fasting that will help you get back control over your body and enjoy the sound of your golden years.

1.1 What Is Intermittent Fasting?

Intermittent fasting is an eating pattern through which you cycle between eating and fasting periods. It doesn't say anything about what things to consume but when to eat them. There are several common sporadic forms of fasting, often splitting the day or week into eating hours and fasting periods.

Every day, most people are already "fast," as they sleep. Intermittent fasting can be as simple as continuing the fast a bit longer. Skip the coffee, eat your first meal at noon, and your last meal at 8 pm. Then you are fasting every day for 16 hours, technically speaking, and limiting your eating to an eating window of 8 hours. This is the most known form of intermittent fasting, called the method 16/8.

Despite what you might think, intermittent fasting is, in fact, very easy to do. Some people report feeling better and having more energy. Hunger is typically not that big of a problem, though it can be a problem at first, as the body gets used to not eating for long periods of time. During the fasting period, no food is allowed, but you can drink water, coffee, tea, and other non-caloric drinks. Some forms of intermittent fasting during the fasting period allow for small amounts of low-calorie foods. You're generally allowed to take supplements while fasting, as long as there are no calories in them.

No. Fasting in one crucial way is different from starvation: control. Deprivation is the unintentional absence of food. This can result in severe pain or even death. On the other hand, fasting is voluntary withholding food for spiritual, health, or other reasons. It is done by someone who is not underweight and therefore has enough body fat stored to live off. Intermittent righteous fasting should not cause suffering, and indeed never death.

Food is easy to get, but you choose not to eat it. This can be for any time, from a few hours to a few days, or even a week or more with medical supervision. You can start a fast at any time of your choice, and you can also end a fast at will. You can start or stop a fast for any reason, or for no reason at all.

Fasting has no traditional length, as it is merely a lack of food. You intermittently fast whenever you are not feeding. For example, the next day, a period of roughly 12-14 hours, you may fast between dinner and breakfast. Intermittent fasting, in that sense, should be considered a part of daily life.

Perhaps it is the oldest and most powerful dietary intervention you can imagine.

Find the word "breakfast". This refers to the meal that breaks your fast-it's done every day. Instead of being some kind of cruel and unusual punishment, the English language simply accepts that fasting should be done every day, even if only for a short period of time.

Intermittent fasting is not an odd and fascinating occurrence, but a part of natural, everyday life.

Why Fasting?

In fact, human beings have been fasting for thousands of years. Sometimes this was done out of desperation when there was practically no food available. It was done in other instances, for religious reasons. Various religions require some sort of fasting, including Islam, Christianity, and Buddhism. Often, also humans and other animals fast instinctively when they are sick.

Clearly, fasting is not "unnatural," and our bodies are very well equipped to handle extended periods of not feeding. All sorts of processes shift in the body when we don't eat for a while, to allow our bodies to survive during a time of famine. It's about hormones, chromosomes, and essential mechanisms of cellular repair.

Once fasted, we get significant decreases in blood sugar and insulin levels, as well as a dramatic rise in human growth hormone. To lose weight, many people do intermittent fasting as it is a straightforward and effective way to limit calories and burn fat. Others do this for the purpose of metabolic health since it can improve different risk factors and health markers.

There is also some evidence that you can be improved by intermittent fasting. Rodent studies show that it can prolong the lifespan as effectively as caps on calories. Some evidence also indicates it can help protect against diseases such as heart disease, type 2 diabetes, cancer, Alzheimer's disease, and others.

It's an easy "life hack" that simplifies your life, while at the same time improving your health. The less you need to plan for the meals, the simpler your life will be.

It also saves time not having to eat 3-4 + times a day (with the preparation and cleaning involved). Much of it.

Do you have to try it?

Intermittent fasting isn't something anyone should do. It's just one of a variety of lifestyle approaches that can improve your health. Still, the most important factors to focus on are eating real food, exercising, and taking care of your sleep.

If you don't like the concept of fasting, then this book can be safely ignored, and you can continue to do what works for you. At the day end, when it comes to nutrition, there is no one-size-fits-all approach. To you, the best diet is the one you can stick to in the long run.

For some people, intermittent fasting is perfect, not others. The only way you can figure out which group you belong to is to try. When you feel good at fasting and consider it a healthy way to eat, it can be a potent tool for weight loss and health enhancement.

Intermittent fasting is not a diet; it is a food pattern. It is a way to plan your meals, so you get the most out of them. Intermittent fasting doesn't affect what you eat; what you eat does.

Why Is It Worth Changing When You're Eating?

Okay, most importantly, without going on a crazy diet or eating your calories down to nothing, it is a great way to get lean. In fact, most of the time, when you start intermittent fasting, you'll try to keep your calories the same. (Most people eat more substantial meals in a shorter timeframe.) However, intermittent fasting is an excellent way to keep the muscle mass on while leaning.

With everything that has been said, the main reason people try intermittent fasting is to lose fat. We're going to talk about how short fasts, in a moment, contribute to fat loss.

Intermittent fasting is one of the most straightforward strategies we have to take off bad weight while maintaining a proper weight since it requires very little change in behavior. This is a perfect thing because it means intermittent fasting falls into the category of "easy enough to do it, but significant enough to make a difference."

How Does Intermittent Fasting Work?

To understand how intermittent fasting contributes to fat loss, we must first understand the difference between fed and fasted state. When it digests and absorbs food, the body is in a fed state. Typically, when you start eating, the fed state starts and lasts three to five hours as your body digests and absorbs the food you just ate. It is challenging for your body to burn fat when you are in the fed condition because your insulin levels are high.

The body goes into what is known as the post-absorptive state after that period of time, which is just a fancy way of saying that your body is not consuming a meal. The post-absorptive condition lasts for 8 to 12 hours after your last meal, which is when you get to the fasted phase. Burning fat in the fasted state is much better for your body because your insulin levels are low. When you're in a fasted state, your body will burn inaccessible fat during the fed state.

Because we are not entering the fasted state until 12 hours after our last meal, it is rare for our bodies to be in this state of fat burning. That is one of the reasons why many people who begin intermittent fasting lose fat without changing what they eat, how much they eat, or how often they exercise. Fasting puts your body in a state of fat burning, which you rarely do during a regular eating schedule.

1.2 Intermittent Fasting for Women Over 50

Some things that make weight loss more difficult after age 50 include decreased appetite, achy joints, and reduced muscle mass, and even sleep problems. At the same time, losing fat, particularly dangerous belly fat, can dramatically reduce your risk for serious health problems such as diabetes, heart attacks, and cancer.

Naturally, the risk of developing many diseases increases as you age. In some cases, intermittent fasting may be functioning as a virtual youth fountain for women over 50, when it comes to weight loss and reducing the chance of usually developing age-related diseases.

Intermittent fasting, often called IF, won't force you to starve. It also does not give you a license to eat lots of unhealthy food during the time you're not fasting. Instead of eating all-day meals and snacks, you're eating within a specific time window.

Most people make an IF schedule, which requires fasting for 12 to 16 hours a day. They eat healthy meals and snacks throughout the rest of the time. You're also allowed to enjoy zero-calorie beverages, such as soda, tea, and coffee.

You will build an eating schedule that will work for the best intermittent fasting outcomes for you. For example:

- **Twelve-hour fasts**: Simply skip breakfast with a 12-12 fast and wait for lunch. If you prefer to eat your meal in the morning, you can eat an early supper and avoid snacks at night. Older women find it rather easy to stick to a 12-12 fast.

- **Seventeen-hour fasts**: With a 16-8 IF cycle, you will enjoy quicker results. Most people choose to eat two meals within an eight-hour window, and a snack or two a day. For example, between noon and eight in the evening, or between eight in the morning and four in the afternoon, you might set your eating time.

- **Five-two schedules:** Limited eating times does not work daily for you. One option is to fast for five days, stick to a twelve-or sixteen-hour plan, and then relax for two days. You could use IF during the week, for example, and usually eat on the weekend.

Another option requires very few calories on alternating days. For instance, on one day, you could keep your calories below 500 and then eat usually the next day.

Remember that frequent IF fasts never claim a low-calorie restriction.

As with any diet, if you're consistent, you'll get the best results. At the same time, on special occasions, you should definitely give yourself a break from this kind of eating routine. To find out which type of intermittent fasting works best for you, you can experiment. With the 12-12 plan, lots of people ease themselves into IF, and then they advance to 16-8. You should later try to stick to that strategy as much as you can.

What Makes Fasting Work Intermittent?

Some people think IF works for them simply because of the limited eating window; of course, it helps them to reduce the number of calories they consume. Instead of consuming three meals and two snacks, for instance, they may find they only have room for two meals and one snack. We become more mindful of the types of food we consume and tend to stay away from processed carbs, unhealthy fat, and empty calories.

You can, of course, choose the kinds of healthy food you love too. While some people opt to decrease their total intake of calories, some combine IF with keno, vegan, or another diet.

Intermittent Fasting Benefits for Women May Extend Beyond Calorie Restriction

Although some nutrition experts argue that IF works only because it naturally helps people to limit their intake of food, others disagree. They believe intermittent fasting results with the same amount of calories and other nutrients are better than typical meal schedules. Reports have even shown that abstaining from food is more than just limiting the number of calories you consume for several hours a day.

These are some of the metabolic changes that IF induces which could help to account for synergistic benefits:

- **Insulin:** Lower insulin levels can help improve fat burning during the fasting period.

- **HGH:** HGH levels rise while insulin levels drop to promote fat burning and muscle growth.

- **Noradrenaline:** The nervous system will send this chemical to the cells in reaction to an empty belly to let them know they need to release fat for fuel.

Is Intermittent Fasting Healthy?

Is intermittent fasting safe? Remember, you're only expected to run for twelve to sixteen hours and not at a time for days. There's still plenty of time to enjoy a balanced, fulfilling diet. Certain older women may need to eat frequently due to metabolic disorders or prescription instructions, of course. In that situation, you can speak to your health care provider about your eating habits before making any changes.

Although it is not actually fasting, during the fasting period, some doctors reported intermittent fasting benefits by having such easy-to-digest foods as whole fruit. Changes like these can still provide needed rest for your digestive and metabolic system. For example, *Fit for Life* was a popular book on weight loss, which suggested eating fruit only after supper and before lunch.

In fact, the writers of this book said they had patients with this twelve-to seventeen-hour "apple" fast each day that just changed their eating habits. We didn't follow the other rules of the diet or count calories, and they still lost weight and became healthier. This strategy could have worked simply because the dieters replaced junk food with whole foods. People found this dietary change to be active and accessible to make anyway. Traditionalists won't call this fasting, but it's essential to know that if you can't absolutely abstain from food for several hours at a time, you may have options.

Typical Intermittent Fasting Results

Doctors and fitness consultant over 50 say it's hard to find any IF downsides in the medical literature. They explained that your blood sugar and insulin level would go down to low levels during the fasting period. Without the hormonal fat-storing signal of insulin, your body will rely on energy for stored fat.

You can also find an overview published by the National Library of Medicine of the intermittent results related to women's health. Some of this report's highlights include studies on using fasting as a tool to reduce the risk of cancer, diabetes, and other metabolic diseases, as well as heart disease.

Is Intermittent Fasting for You the Best Fat-Loss Tool?

In any case, IF seems to work mostly because people find adherence reasonably easy. We say it helps them to reduce calories naturally and make better food choices by reducing the amount of food they eat. Many studies suggest IF is better than just cutting calories, carbohydrates, or fat because it seems to encourage fat loss while maintaining lean muscle mass.

Obviously, most people use IF with a different weight-loss strategy. For example, you might decide to lose weight by eating 1,200 calories a day. With two meals and two snacks, you can find it much easier to spread 1,200 calories than in three meals and three snacks. If you've been struggling with weight loss because either your diet didn't work or was just too hard to stick to, you could try intermittent fasting for quicker results.

Chapter 2: Types of Intermittent Fasting

Intermittent fasting has been very trendy in recent years. It is claimed to cause weight loss, improve metabolic health, and maybe even extend lifespan. Given the popularity, it is not surprising that several different types or methods of intermittent fasting were created. Every type can be useful, but it depends on the individual to figure out which one works best.

THE 16/8 METHOD

	DAY 1	DAY 2	DAY 3	DAY 4	DAY 5	DAY 6	DAY 7
Midnight / 4 AM / 8 AM	FAST	FAST	FAST	FAST	FAST	FAST	FAST
12 PM	First meal	First meal	First meal	First meal	First meal	First meal	First meal
4 PM	Last meal by 8pm	Last meal by 8pm	Last meal by 8pm	Last meal by 8pm	Last meal by 8pm	Last meal by 8pm	Last meal by 8pm
8 PM / Midnight	FAST	FAST	FAST	FAST	FAST	FAST	FAST

Here are six popular ways to practice intermittent fasting.

1. The 16/8 Methods: Fast for 16 Hours a Day:

The 16/8 Method involves fasting for 14 to16 hours a day and reducing the "food period" –8-10 hours a day. In the eating cycle, you can fit for 2, 3, or more meals.

Also known as the Leangains Protocol, this method has been popularized by fitness expert Martin Berkhan. Just making this fasting approach can be as easy as not eating anything after dinner and skipping breakfast.

If you end your last meal at 8 p.m., for example, and don't eat until noon the next day, you have been fasting for 16 hours, technically. It is generally recommended that women fast just 14-15 hours, because, with slightly shorter fasts, they seem to do better.

This method is popular since most people are already fasting while they're sleeping. It is convenient as you quickly prolong the overnight by skipping breakfast and not eating until lunch. Some of the most common approaches?

System 16/8: Lunch only by 11 a.m. And 7:00 p.m. And morning, and 8 p.m.

System 14/10: Meal only by 10 a.m. And 8:00 p.m.

It may take a few days to find the right eating and fasting windows for this process, mainly if you are very busy or if you wake up hungry for breakfast. This method may be difficult to get used to at first for people who get hungry in the morning and like to eat breakfast. A lot of breakfast-skippers actually eat this way naturally, though. During the fast, you can drink water, coffee, and other non-caloric drinks, which can help to reduce hunger feelings.

Mostly eating healthy foods is very important during your eating time. This method won't work if you're eating lots of junk food or too many calories. When you start your eating time of 8–hour, it doesn't matter. Beginning at 8 am and ending at 4 pm. Or you will start at 2 pm and then stop at 10 pm. Do whatever you want to do. I tend to find that eating around 1 pm and 8 pm works well because I can eat lunch and dinner with friends and family at those times.

Because intermittent daily fasting is performed on this schedule, it becomes straightforward to get into the habit of eating. You're probably eating about the same time each day right now, without thinking about it. Okay, it's the same thing with regular intermittent fasting; just learn not to eat at certain hours, which is remarkably easy.

One potential disadvantage of this schedule is that because you typically cut out one or two meals out of your day, getting the same number of calories over the week becomes more difficult. Simply put, it's tough to teach yourself to eat larger meals consistently. The result is that lots of people who try this intermittent fasting style end up losing weight. That can be either a good thing or a bad thing, depending on your objectives.

2. The Diet of 5:2: Fast 2 Days a Week

The diet of 5:2 or fast food involves eating 500-600 calories for two days a week and regularly eating the remaining 5 days.

This approach to IF focuses on two days a week, capping your calories at 500. You maintain a healthy and regular diet during the other 5 days of the week.

This method usually includes a 200-calorie meal and a 300-calorie meal on days of fasting. Focusing on high-fiber and high-protein foods is essential in order to help fill you up but also to keep low calories while fasting.

You can choose which two days of fasting (say, Tuesdays and Thursdays) as long as there is between them a day of no-fasting.

Avoid eating the same amount of food you would normally eat on non-fasting days.

This diet is also called The Easy Diet and was popularized by Michael Mosley, a British journalist. It is recommended on the days of fasting that women eat 500 calories and that men eat 600 calories.

You might generally eat every day of the week except Mondays and Thursdays, for example. You eat two small meals for those two days (250 calories per women's meal, and 300 calories for men).

As the critics correctly point out, there are no studies evaluating the 5:2 diet itself, but there are many reports on the effects of intermittent fasting.

3. Eat-Stop-Eat: Do a Fast 24 Hour, Once or Twice A Week:

This method involves a 24-hour rapid complete. Also, it occurs just once or twice a week. From breakfast to snack, or lunch to lunch, most people fast. With this IF version, the side effects, such as fatigue, headaches, irritability, hunger, and low energy, can be extreme.

When you follow this process, then on your non-fasting days, you can return to a regular, healthy diet. This technique was popularized by Brad Pylon, a fitness expert, and has been popular for some years.

If you end dinner, for example, at 7 p.m. Monday and don't have dinner until 7 p.m., you just did a full24-hour fast the next day.

EAT-STOP-EAT

DAY 1	DAY 2	DAY 3	DAY 4	DAY 5	DAY 6	DAY 7
Eats normally	24-hour fast	Eats normally	Eats normally	24-hour fast	Eats normally	Eats normally

You can fast from breakfast to breakfast, or from lunch to lunch as well. The end result is close. During the fast, tea, coffee, and other non-caloric beverages are allowed, but no solid foods are allowed.

If you do this to lose weight, it is essential that you usually eat during the times of fasting. As in, eat as much food as if you hadn't been fasting anyway. The potential downside of this approach is that a lot of people will consider an easy, relatively troublesome 24-hour complete.

You don't need to go all - in straight away, though. It's a good beginning with 14-16 hours, and then moving up from there.

Perhaps the most significant advantage of doing a 24-hour fast is getting over the fasting mental barrier. If you've never fasted before, finishing your first one successfully makes you know you're not going to die if you don't eat for a day.

ALTERNATE-DAY FASTING

DAY 1	DAY 2	DAY 3	DAY 4	DAY 5	DAY 6	DAY 7
Eats normally	24-hour fast OR Eat only a few hundred calories	Eats normally	24-hour fast OR Eat only a few hundred calories	Eats normally	24-hour fast OR Eat only a few hundred calories	Eats normally

4.   **Alternate-Day Fasting: Fast Every Other Day**:

Alternate-day fasting means fasting every other day. Various versions of this method are available. Some of them allow fasting days to be around 500 calories. Many of the laboratory studies that demonstrated the health benefits of intermittent fasting used some version of this method.

Reduce your calories to 500 or around 25 percent of your regular intake on fasting days, for example. Resume your daily, healthy diet on days of no-fasting. (There are also stringent variations in this approach which include consuming 0 calories on alternative days instead of 500.)

Interesting note: One study showed that people following this IF pattern had significantly increased levels of LDL (or bad) cholesterol for six months after another six months off the diet. Every other day, a complete fast can seem slightly extreme, so it's not recommended for beginners. With this method, several times a week, you'll be going to bed very hungry, which is not very pleasant and probably unsustainable in the long run.

The advantage of intermittent alternating day fasting is that it gives you a long time in the fasted state than the fasting style of Leangains. That would hypothetically increase the benefits of fasting.

Yet, in practice, you may be able to feast for a meal, but preparing to do so every day of the week takes a little preparation, plenty of cooking, and good food. The end result is that most people who try intermittent fasting end up losing some weight because their meals remain similar in size even though a few snacks are cut out every week.

If you're looking to lose weight, that's not an issue. And even if you're happy with your weight, if you follow the daily fasting schedules or the weekly fasting schedules, this won't prove too much of a problem. However, if you fast on multiple days a week for 24 hours a day, then it will be challenging to eat enough of your festive days to make up for that.

As a result, it's a better idea to try intermittent fasting on a daily basis or fast a single 24 hours once a week or once a month.

5. The Warrior Diet: Eat a Huge Meal at Night:

The Warrior Diet was popularized by the fitness expert Ori Hofmekler, fast during the day. During the day, it involves eating small quantities of raw fruits and vegetables and eating one massive meal at night.

Basically, within a 4-hour eating window, you "fast" the entire day and "feast" the night.

One of the most popular "diets" to include some form of intermittent fasting was the Warrior Diet. This diet also highlights food choices that are quite similar to a whole, unprocessed, pale diet that resembles what they looked like in nature.

THE WARRIOR DIET

	DAY 1	DAY 2	DAY 3	DAY 4	DAY 5	DAY 6	DAY 7
Midnight 4 AM 8 AM 12 PM	Eating only small amounts of vegetables and fruits	Eating only small amounts of vegetables and fruits	Eating only small amounts of vegetables and fruits	Eating only small amounts of vegetables and fruits	Eating only small amounts of vegetables and fruits	Eating only small amounts of vegetables and fruits	Eating only small amounts of vegetables and fruits
4 PM	Large meal	Large meal	Large meal	Large meal	Large meal	Large meal	Large meal
8 PM Midnight							

6. Skip Meals When Convenient:

You don't really have to pursue a formal intermittent fasting program to enjoy some of the benefits. Another choice is to actually skip meals from time to time, like when you're not feeling hungry or being too busy to cook and then eat.

It's a myth that people need to eat every couple of hours, or hit "starvation mode" or lose muscle. The human body is well-equipped to handle long periods of drought, let alone losing from time to time a meal or two.

SPONTANEOUS MEAL SKIPPING

DAY 1	DAY 2	DAY 3	DAY 4	DAY 5	DAY 6	DAY 7
Breakfast	Skipped Meal	Breakfast	Breakfast	Breakfast	Breakfast	Breakfast
Lunch	Lunch	Lunch	Lunch	Lunch	Lunch	Lunch
Dinner	Dinner	Dinner	Dinner	Skipped Meal	Dinner	Dinner

So, if one day you're not really hungry, skip breakfast and eat a healthy lunch and dinner. And, if you're traveling somewhere, and you can't find anything you'd like to eat, do a short fast.

When you feel inclined to do so, skipping, one or two meals, is essentially a spontaneous sporadic, fast. Just make sure the rest of the people are eating healthy foods.

The Bottom Line:

A lot of people with some of these methods are getting great results. Not everybody gets intermittent fasting. It is not something that anybody has to do. It is just another tool in the toolbox that some people may find useful.

Many people also think that women might not profit as much as men. It may also not be a healthy choice for people who have or are vulnerable to eating disorders.

Remember to eat safely, too, if you decide to try intermittent fasting. During the eating periods, it is not possible to binge on junk food and expect to lose weight and improve health. Calories still count, and food quality remains important.

Chapter 3: Benefits and Risks of Intermittent Fasting

Intermittent fasting has become a prevalent phenomenon among celebrities, non-eaters, and others, a diet plan that oscillates between specified eating and non-eating cycles.

While intermittent fasting benefits are still being researched, there is evidence that the practice has adverse side effects such as hair loss, anxiety, and stress. Such signs could be an indication that your diet is about to stop. In this chapter, we describe the benefits and risk of intermittent fasting and help you to choose the best way.

3.1 Is Intermittent Fasting for Everyone?

Intermittent fasting is not for everyone. It's another tool to have in your toolkit for individuals who have struggled to lose weight. In the end, it's about the lifestyle of a person and the choices they make. They've got to weigh the options and decide, "What's going to work for me?"

Intermittent fasting offers a number of benefits for the body. Numerous studies have shown that the eating plan could help people increase stress tolerance, raise blood sugar levels, and decrease blood pressure and heart rate resting.

Fasting causes changes in metabolism in the way people respond to food shortages. When the body uses sugar reserves to skip meals for specific periods of time, and transforms fats into energy, a new study shows that there are two forms of fasting that cause positive changes in the body. One is limiting feeding to six to eight hours a day, and the other is reducing food to two days a week for another moderate-sized meal.

According to a study co-author and a professor of neuroscience at the School of Medicine, the two eating patterns may help people better manage blood lipid levels, increase their resting heart rates, avoid stress and maintain proper blood sugar levels and blood pressure.

We are at a transition point where we could soon consider adding intermittent fasting knowledge to medical school curricula alongside regular healthy diet and exercise guidance. The thesis underpinned the results of earlier human and animal studies. Intermittent fasting also causes the same changes in animals' metabolism and improves their behavior and DNA, according to Gerald Bernstein, program coordinator at the

Lenox Hill Hospital's Friedman Diabetes Institute in New York City.

Certain animal studies have shown that intermittent fasting can delay the growth of cancer tumors and Alzheimer's disease. A health expert, however, cautioned that not every person might enjoy the health benefits of fasting. There are some groups of people that should avoid having meals missed.

"Intermittent fasting may not be a good diet on medications and/or insulin for diabetic patients that could have swings in blood sugar," he said. "Intermittent fasting is not for older patients. It is necessary to watch for hypoglycemia, which can lead to falls."

First of all, intermittent fasting isn't just another way to say "free ride." Randomly skipping meals while still eating a diet high in processed foods won't help you lose fat or improve your health. So while there is no "right" way to practice fasting, a certain amount of attention to nutritional detail will be required in any proper procedure. You got to be ready to do that task.

Some will consider IF too painful or uncomfortable to exercise. And for others, any future benefits far outweigh its risks. Perhaps IF could be quite risky for some people. You probably want to know before you miss your next meal if you fall into that category.

Here is the lowdown, based on numerous case studies and a limited amount of research written:

Intermittent Fasting: Green Light

You are most likely to be successful with intermittent fasting if:

• You have a history of controlling calorie and food intake (e.g., you've "died" before)

• You're already an accomplished exerciser

• You're single, or you don't have children

• Your spouse (if you have one) is incredibly supportive

• Your job allows you to have low-perfection times

Intermittent fasting: Yellow Light:

In the meantime, if you meet the following requirements, you may want to proceed with caution:

• You are married or have children

• You have performance-oriented or customer-oriented jobs

• You participate in sport/athletics

• You are female

Again, the first three factors make it much more difficult to obey IF guidelines and may make it impossible for you to do so. What's more, trying to fast can conflict with your sport's performance goals.

As for the last case, some experimenters say that for women, fasting induces sleeplessness, anxiety, irregular periods, and other hormone dysregulation signs. Especially in the stricter forms of intermittent fasting, women seem to fare worse than men do.

Intermittent Fasting: Red Light:

Finally, some people are not really supposed to bother about intermittent fasting. Don't try it if:

• You're pregnant

• You have a history of disordered eating

• You're chronically stressed

• You're not sleeping well

• You're new to diet and exercise

If you're new to diet and exercise, intermittent fasting may look like a magic weight loss bullet. But before you start experimenting with fasts, it would be a lot smarter to fix any nutritional deficiencies. First, make sure you start from a stable nutritional platform.

Pregnant women have increased energy needs, so this is not the time to fast if you start a family. Ditto if you have chronic stress and/or are not sleeping. Your body needs to be nurtured, not extra weight.

And if you've struggled in the past with disordered eating, you're likely to recognize that a fasting protocol could lead you down a path that could cause you more problems.

3.2 Benefits or Advantages of Intermittent Fasting

Nutrition is fuel. As we feed, insulin levels increase, converting sugar in the blood into energy and helping the body store any glucose we don't need immediately. For fast access, we store about a day's worth of power in the liver and muscles. Anything extra is fat.

When we do not eat for a while, our bodies break down the energy stored for fuel. That is behind intermittent fasting theory.

Go without eating for long enough, and you will start burning fat. That's why the emphasis with intermittent fasting is less on what you eat, and move on when you eat.

We seem to eat all the time right now. According to the study, 67 percent of eating between meals occurs in Canada. It says that these habits evolved due, in part, to the erroneous belief that regular, smaller meals would improve metabolism and help with weight loss. Constant snacking actually keeps the insulin levels elevated, increasing the risk of insulin resistance.

Health Benefits of Intermittent Fasting

It makes sense that less caloric intake consumption would help you lose weight. Fasting, however, is not the same as hunger. This means the length of feeding is shortened, but the number of nutrients and the daily caloric requirements are still being met.

We had to eat and engage in intermittent fasting during an eight-hour window in a study involving 24 participants. During the intermittent fasting timeframe, participants were evaluated with weight training, and calories were ingested. It was concluded that their lean mass was significant in resting energy expenditure from the first day until the last. Intermittent fasting, together with resistance training, will minimize body fat and improve body composition.

The most obvious benefit of intermittent fasting is weight loss. There are, however, other potential advantages beyond this, some of which have been recognized since ancient times.

The fasting cycles were often referred to as 'cleanses,' 'detoxifications,' or ' purifications,' but the concept is identical–for example, abstaining from eating food for some time, often for health reasons. People imagined that this time of food abstinence would remove and rejuvenate toxin systems in their bodies. They were perhaps more right than they understood.

Some of the alleged health benefits of intermittent fasting include:

- Weight and body fat reduction

- Increased fat burning

- Lower blood insulin and sugar levels

- Possible reversal of type 2 diabetes

- Probably improved mental focus and concentration

- Possibly increased energy

- Likely increased growth hormone, at least in the short term

- Perhaps improved blood cholesterol profile

While diets can complicate life, it may be simplified with intermittent fasting. While foods can be costly, it can be free to fast intermittently. Fasting is possible anywhere where diets may be limited in their availability. And as discussed earlier, fasting is a potentially powerful way to lower insulin and lower body weight.

Here, we briefly explain some evidence-based benefits of intermittent fasting:

1. Intermittent fasting changes the role of cells, genes, and hormones:

When you're not eating for a while, there are several things in your body that happen. For example, your body starts critical processes of cellular repair and changes the hormone levels, so that stored body fat is more accessible.

Here are some of the changes that take place in your body during fasting:

• **Insulin levels:** Insulin levels drop dramatically in the blood, which promotes fat burning.

• **Human growth hormone**: Growth hormone blood levels can increase up to 5-fold. Higher levels of this hormone help in burning fat and gaining muscle, and have many other benefits.

• **Cellular repair:** The body causes essential processes of cellular repairs, such as removing waste material from cells.

• **Gene expression:** Different genes and molecules have beneficial effects related to survival and disease prevention.

These changes in hormones, gene expression, and cell function are linked to many of the advantages of intermittent fasting.

2. Intermittent fasting helps you lose weight and abdominal fat

Many who seek intermittent fasting do it to lose weight. The intermittent fasting would usually make you eat fewer meals. Unless you make up for it by eating much more during the other meals, you will end up taking fewer calories. Therefore, intermittent fasting improves hormone regulation to reduce weight loss.

Lower levels of insulin, higher levels of growth hormone, and elevated concentrations of norepinephrine (noradrenaline) all increase body fat breakdown and promote its energy usage.

In fact, short-term fasting increases your metabolic rate by 3.6-14 percent, which helps you burn even more calories. Intermittent fasting, in other words, operates on both sides of the calorie equation. This increases your metabolic rate and reduces the amount of food you eat (reduces calories in).

According to a 2014 scientific literature analysis, intermittent fasting can cause weight loss of 3-8 percent over 3-24 weeks. That is a huge amount. People have lost 4-7 percent of their waist circumference, meaning they lost lots of belly fat, the unhealthy fat that causes disease in the abdominal cavity.

One research study also showed that intermittent fasting resulted in less muscle loss than a prolonged limit on calories. Despite everything, intermittent fasting can be an incredibly powerful tool for weight loss.

3.	**Intermittent fasting can reduce insulin resistance and your risk of type 2 diabetes**:

Type 2 diabetes in recent decades has become incredibly common. Its main feature in terms of insulin resistance is high blood sugar levels.

Anything that reduces insulin resistance would help lower blood sugar levels and safeguard against type 2 diabetes. Ironically, it has been shown that intermittent fasting has significant benefits for insulin resistance, contributing to a remarkable reduction in blood sugar.

Studies on intermittent fasting show while fasting insulin has been reduced by 20-31%. Only one study in diabetic rats found that intermittent fasting protected against kidney damage, one of the most severe diabetes complications. What this means is that intermittent fasting for people at risk of developing type 2 diabetes can be highly protective.

There can be some variations between genders, however. One female study showed that blood sugar control actually worsened after an intermittent fasting protocol that lasted for 22 days.

4. Intermittent fasting in the body will reduce oxidizing stress and inflammation:

Oxidative stress is one of the aging and many chronic diseases. This includes unstable molecules, called free radicals, which react to other essential molecules (such as protein and DNA) and cause damage. Many studies show that intermittent fasting can improve the body's oxidative stress resistance.

Additionally, studies show intermittent fasting can help fight inflammation, another key driver of common diseases of all kinds.

5. Intermittent fasting can benefit health for heart:

Currently, heart disease is a giant killer in the world. It is known that different health markers (so-called "risk factors") are associated with either increased or decreased risk of heart disease.

Numerous different risk factors have been shown to boost intermittent fasting, including blood pressure, HDL and LDL cholesterol, blood triglycerides, inflammatory markers, and blood sugar levels. Much of this is, however, based on animal research. There is a need to study the effects on heart health much further in humans before recommendations can be made.

6. Intermittent Fasting induces a number of cellular repair processes:

When we fast, the cells in the body initiate a cellular process of "waste removal," called autophagy. It involves breaking down the cells and metabolizing the damaged and defective proteins that, over time, build up inside the cells. Enhanced autophagy can provide protection against a variety of illnesses, including cancer and Alzheimer's.

7. Intermittent fasting can help prevent cancer:

Cancer is a terrible disease with uncontrolled cell growth. Fasting has been shown to have some beneficial effects on metabolism, which could lead to reduced cancer risk.

Given the need for human studies, promising evidence from animal studies suggests that intermittent fasting may help to prevent cancer. There is also some evidence for patients with human cancer, which shows that fasting has reduced various side effects of chemotherapy.

8. Intermittent fasting is right for your brain:

 What's right for your body is good for your mind too. Intermittent fasting improves the different metabolic features that are considered to be critical for brain health. It involves reduced oxidative stress, decreased inflammation, and decreasing levels of blood sugar and insulin resistance.

Several rat studies have shown that intermittent fasting can boost the growth of new nerve cells, which should benefit brain function. It also raises brain hormone levels called brain-derived neurotropic factor (BDNF), a deficit affecting depression, and many other brain issues. Animal studies have shown that sporadic stroke-fasting protects against brain damage.

9. Intermittent fasting may help with prevention of Alzheimer's disease:

Alzheimer's disease is the most common neurodegenerative disease in the world. There is no treatment available for Alzheimer's, so it is essential to keep it from occurring in the first place.

A rat study showed intermittent fasting could delay the onset of Alzheimer's disease or decrease its severity. In a series of reports, a lifestyle change involving regular short-term fasts could significantly improve the symptoms of Alzheimer's in 9 out of 10 patients. Animal studies also suggest that fasting can protect against other neurodegenerative diseases, including disease caused by Parkinson and Huntington.

10. Intermittent fasting can prolong your lifespan, help you live longer:

One of the intermittent fasting's most exciting applications may be its ability to extend the lifespan.

Studies in rats showed that intermittent fasting improves lifespan similarly to constant calorie restriction. The effects had been quite dramatic in some of these studies. In one of them, rats who fasted every other day lived 83 percent longer than non-fasted rats.

While this is far from being proved in humans, intermittent fasting among the anti-aging crowd has become very common.

Given the known metabolism benefits and all sorts of health markers, it makes sense that intermittent fasting would help you live longer, healthier lives.

The Practical Benefits of Intermittent Fasting

Low-carb high-fat (LCHF) foods are effective for weight loss, but by incorporating intermittent fasting, which provides many benefits not offered by traditional nutrition, we can theoretically do even better. All diets have the same aims, which are to enhance metabolic health, reduce the effect of insulin, and increase the loss of weight. While many agree that weight gain is caused by excess calories alone, that is only partial. Calories and insulin are both likely to drive weight gain. LCHF diets decrease insulin, regardless of calories, but typically still reduce calories without even trying. Hence, LCHF is impressively effective for weight loss. The combination of fasting and LCHF, however, could have a synergistic advantage for maximum effect.

1. Cheap:

Simply put, some people can't afford the good to eat. How is it that fresh cherries cost $6.99/pound, and will cost $1.99 to buy a whole loaf of bread? Buying pasta and white bread is a lot easier to feed a family on a budget.

But that doesn't mean they should be doomed to type 2 diabetes and disability for a lifetime. Fasting is gratis. It's not just free actually, but it actually saves money because you don't need to buy any food. Nothing beats free, except to save money, of course. Who cannot use some extra dollars in their wallet when losing weight and, at the same time, being healthier? It's like you get paid for weight loss!

2. Convenience:

Having a home-cooked, scratch-cooked meal is excellent, but there are many people who simply don't have the time or the inclination to do so. Over the last some decades, the number of meals consumed away from home has increased. While there are many who try to support the 'slow food' movement, it's evident that the idea is resisted by modern society.

Don't get it wrong; maybe you like to cook as much as the next guy does, butut it takes just a lot of time. It just doesn't leave much time between work and getting kids to school stuff and hockey.

And asking people to dedicate themselves, as noble as it may be, to home cooking isn't a winning strategy for some. Fasting is the same, on the other hand. You save time because you don't have time to buy food, shop, cook and clean. It's a way to simplify your life. Where many diets make your life more complicated (eat this, but not that, and just a little of the other), it's more straightforward with fasting. You save time, and you save money. It just is not getting any better.

3. Cheat days:

Is it realistic to encourage people to eat ice cream ever again? Live for life? It's a long time forever, and celebrations are happening. You can't eat dessert every single day, but fasting gives some of the ability to enjoy that dessert from time to time because, by fasting, you can balance the scales if you feast.

Cheat days are important because they can help build compliance for the other days for some people. While others may do best with an all-or-none approach, fasting may help balance the "cheat" days for those who struggle with it forever. The critical aspect of fasting is incorporating it into your life. Please note that we are not recommending a "binge," followed by a fast "punish" on yourself. Instead, we feel some people are going to do better with an occasional treat they can match with a fast. Life is fleeting. Good days and bad days are over. There are days for celebrating and days for dreading. It is life. Not all, but some people may also benefit from intermittent diets.

4. Power:

Hard to lose weight. Anyone knows it. This is the most critical issue of any dietary plan-is, is it going to work? The calorie reduction diet eat-less, move-more sounds like it should work, but does it actually work? The response for most people is no.

For some people, some diets work enormously but fail utterly for others. Diets often operate for a period of time and then seem to be stalling.

Fasting is almost universally effective, as it is the fastest and most efficient way of reducing insulin. It also contains practically unlimited power. What are we talking about? Many diets have only 1 setting for the 'strength.' If you follow the diet of the Mediterranean but do not lose weight, then what? How are you becoming more 'Mediterranean'? There is only one power mode, and either it is working, or it is not so fasting. You can fast for 10 hours or 10 days (although we do not recommend prolonged fasts on a routine basis, and if you choose to do one, please ensure that it is with medical care).

You have to ask yourself this question: Would you think you lose weight if you don't eat anything for 1 week? Even a kid knows you've got to lose weight. Nearly unavoidable.

Just two outstanding questions remain. First of all-Is this unhealthy? On the contrary, the potential health benefits are substantial. Three, would you? Okay, you'll never know if you've never done it. We assume that almost everyone can do that.

5. Flexibility

Fasting can be performed every time, wherever. If for whatever reason, you're not feeling good, you just stop. It is completely reversible in minutes. Consider bariatric surgery (stapling to the stomach). Such operations are carried out in such a way that people can fast for extended periods of time. In the short term, at least, they tend to work. But there are significant potential risks in these surgeries, almost all of which are irreversible.

There is no defined length. For 16 hours or 16 days, you can fast. No schedule is set. This week, you can fast a lot, and next week, none. It can change with the timetable of your life. You may fast for any reason or for no reason whatsoever. Therefore, why would we think anyone can't fast for 1 week or one month without having ever done it?

6. Add to any diet:

Here's the most significant benefit of all. Any diet can include intermittent fasting. It is more subtraction than an addition.

- You aren't eating meat? You can still go fast.

- Are you not eating wheat? You can still go fast.

- Are you allergic to nut? You can still do it quickly.

- Don't you have time? You can still go fast.

- Do you have no money? You can still go fast.

- All the time you're traveling? You can still go fast.

- Don't you cook? You can still go fast.

- Are you 80 years old? You can still go fast.

- Do you have the chewing or swallowing problems? You can still go fast.

Just. Easy. What better way than that? Choose your best accordingly.

3.3 Risks or Disadvantages of Intermittent Fasting

Fasting is a practice, but intermittent fasting, a diet plan that oscillates between specified eating and not eating cycles, only recently became ultra-popular following slew endorsements from celebrities and tech moguls.

Fasting enthusiasts say that helps with concentration, loss of weight, and energy. Yet intermittent fasting, like any diet, can cause severe eating habits. The adverse side effects of fasting might, in some cases, outweigh any potential benefit. Here are some signs an irregular pattern of fasting is dangerous or harmful.

- **Intermittent Fasting Will Interfere with Your Sleep, Which Is Important to Your Health:**

There is some preliminary evidence that intermittent fasting may boost sleep by preventing you from waking up in the middle of the night. If people start their fast earlier, they also appear to close their eating window well before going to bed. This helps them avoid snacking during the night, which can improve sleep quality.

Yet intermittent fasting can also interfere with your sleep cycle or trigger restless nights. Multiple studies have shown that fasting can reduce your amount of REM sleep, which is thought to improve your memory, mood, and learning ability.

- **It Could Also Make You Less Conscious or Alert:**

Low endurance is another potential side effect of intermittent fasting.

Jack Dorsey believed his fasting diet would keep him more concentrated and alert, but some nutritionists would attribute these feelings to his body going into hunger mode.

Intermittent fasting can lead to reduced alertness in the long term because the body does not eat enough calories during a fasting period to provide sufficient energy. Fasting can also result in fatigue, concentration difficulties, or dizziness.

- **If You Break the Fast Too Early:**

Fasting for longer than 24 hours is considered "extreme"; your diet should not include self-shaming or guilt, but even shorter fasts can have extreme health consequences.

If people give themselves a window of time to eat, they can start feeling guilty of breaking their fast too early or eating too late. Any kind of anxiety or shame that surrounds your diet can be a warning sign of disordered conduct. This involves talking to yourself about another symptom of orthopraxis when you are fasting. Which is defined as an obsession with eating properly or 'healthily.' Symptoms include a constant need to talk about your diet, and a concern about what you're going to eat next.

When you find that your diet has become inflexible so much so that social events are skipped or canceled because they don't suit your eating habits, take heed, and consider moving to another dieting process.

- **Intermittent Fasting Will Raise Cortisol Levels, Leaving You Stressed:**

Because of intermittent fasting, men are less susceptible to elevated cortisol levels than women. Recent research has found that intermittent fasting may reduce the risk of diabetes, cancer, and heart disease, but depriving yourself of food for a prolonged period of time may raise levels of cortisol, the stress hormone of the body.

Especially when you spend more extended periods depriving yourself of food. Cortisol is the stress hormone of the body, and the increased levels are associated with increased stress and accumulation of fat. Even if there are theoretically any positive health effects, the increase in tension will eliminate them. High levels of cortisol are also correlated with fat storage, which is not desirable if you try to lose weight.

- **When You Lose Your Time or Experience Hair Loss, It May Be Linked to Fasting:**

Any diet that leads to a calorie deficit-increasing can cause symptoms such as hair loss or missing period.

Intermittent fasting can cause some people to go into a calorie deficit that can result in hair loss and periods that are irregular or missed. Despite low blood sugar, people on an intermittent fasting diet may also feel colder than usual.

- **Anxiety, Depression, or Antisocial Feelings May Be A Tip-Off that the Diet Is Not Healthy:**

Every type of diet is like hunger. Intermittent fasting transforms into disordered eating when it starts to affect one's wellbeing, which involves a shift in mental and social behavior, such as an increase in anxiety and depression or a decrease in the ability to socialize.

- **If You Feel Hungry, You Might Want to Consider Calling It Quits:**

When it comes to diet, ask yourself: "Is this going to create motherhood?" Usually, you don't advocate any kind of strict fasting outside of that, because what you're doing overrides the body's instincts. Instead, people should listen to the typical signs of their bodies as to whether they're hungry or full.

It is a real thing to get hungry. People can genuinely become irritable.

In Short:

People need fuel to stay healthy, so we should listen to what our bodies need and not build fast and challenging food habits laws.

Although intermittent fasting is not necessarily unhealthy, people with an eating disorder's personal or family background should be steering away from the diet. The method is also not suitable for highly active people because they need more electricity.

Chapter 4: Recommended Food for Intermittent Fasting

While the word "fasting" sounds terrifying, intermittent fasting (IF) takes the diet world by storm. With the right amount of research on the positive impact of the diet on body weight, memory, and blood sugar, it's no wonder that the IF bandwagon seems to be running to everyone you go. Perhaps the appeal is the lack of rules governing food. When you can eat, there are limits but not precisely what you can consume. So should you be downing ice cream pints and chip bags while fasting intermittently? Likely not. That's why we have put together a list of the best foods to be included in your IF life.

If Refresher

We've previously given you the low-down on intermittent fasting, but here's a little refresher. There are multiple IF plans, but most of them focus on fasting in the day or days of the week for a certain number of hours.

Here's a rundown of the most commonly used IF models:

So, What Should We Eat?

There are no requirements or limits on what form or how much food to consume after intermittent fasting. The IF benefits are unlikely to follow regular Big Macs meals; there are entirely different rules for what you can eat and drink, depending on whether you're in your eating period or fasting window.

In fact, you can follow a variety of intermittent fasting schedules. The most **frequent is** the 16/8 plan, which means you're eating for an 8-hour window and 16-hour fast. You can also choose to eat windows shorter or longer, or you may want to fast alternately.

A well-balanced diet is key to weight loss, energy levels, and dietary adherence. Anyone who wishes to lose weight will concentrate on nutrient-dense foods such as vegetables, berries, whole grains, nuts, beans, seeds and milk, and lean proteins. Foods usually suggested for improved health high-fiber, unprocessed, whole foods are offering variety and flavor. In other words, eat plenty of the foods below, and, while fasting, you will not end up in a hanging rage.

1. Water

Although you're not eating, it's essential for so many reasons to stay hydrated, as the health of basically every major organ in your body. The amount of water any person should drink varies, but at all times, you want your urine to be a pale yellow color. Dark yellow urine indicates dehydration that can lead to headaches, tiredness, and light-headedness. Couple that with a limited diet, and it could be a disaster recipe. If you don't get excited by the thought of plain water, add a squeeze of lemon juice, a few mint leaves or slices of cucumber to your water. That is going to be our little secret.

Why Is Water So Valuable?

Staying hydrated helps curb hunger, making it easier to adhere to your fasting diet, but there are many other health benefits as well. Drinking water helps lubricate your joints, controls your body temperature, and ensures a standard digestive system.

Water also brings oxygen and other nutrients into your bodies; flushes waste out of your body and helps keep your blood pressure stable.

Carbonized Water vs. Flavored Water

Carbonated, or seltzer, water is allowed when fasting intermittently; just make sure you are vigilant in reading labels. While there are no added sweeteners to pure seltzer water, some flavored water drinks do, and misunderstanding is easy to have.

Read the list of ingredients and avoid something, such as aspartame or sucralose, with added sugar or artificial sweeteners. Even water flavored with natural sweeteners such as stevia can kick-start a craving for sugar and make it harder for you to stick your fast.

Choose plain seltzer water or seltzer water, which is only flavored with natural flavors or essences of fruit.

Can You Drink Only Water?

While water is supposed to be king when it comes to drinking options, you can also drink black coffee herbal tea. Black coffee will not break your fast or push you out of ketosis. Caffeine may even increase metabolism, thus helping to promote weight loss. Black coffee also helps curb your appetite, which can make it much more manageable to get through your morning quickly.

But it's essential for it to be black. If you add cream, milk, and or sugar to your coffee, you are going to break your fast.

2. Avocado

While consuming the highest calorie fruit when trying to lose weight might seem counterintuitive, the monounsaturated fat in avocado is extremely satiating. One study even found that adding half an avocado to your lunch would keep you full for hours longer than consuming the green gem.

3. Fish

There is a reason for eating at least eight ounces of fish a week in the Dietary Guidelines. It is costly not only in healthy fats and protein, but also contains sufficient amounts of vitamin D. And if you consume only a small amount of food all day long, don't you want one that provides more nutrient bang for your buck? Not to mention that restricting your intake of calories will mess with your cognition, and fish is often considered a "brain food."

4. Cruciferous Veggies

Plants like broccoli, sprouts from Brussels, and cauliflower are all packed with the fiber. Eating fiber-rich foods that keep you healthy and avoid constipation is essential when you eat erratically. Fiber also has the ability to make your stomach feel full, which, if you can't eat again for 16 hours, is something you might want.

5. Potatoes

Repeat after me: "Each white food is not weak."

Case in point: Studies have shown that vegetables are among the most satiating foods available. Another study found potato eating as part of a healthy diet could help with weight loss. Sorry, not counting French fries and potato chips.

5. Beans and Legumes

Your favorite addition to chili on the IF lifestyle, maybe your best friend. Food, especially carbs, provides activity energy. While we're not telling you to carbo-load, throwing some low-calorie carbs, such as beans and legumes, into your eating plan would definitely not hurt. In addition, foods such as chickpeas, black beans, peas, and lentils have been shown to decrease body weight, even without minimal calories.

6. Probiotics

Do you know what you like most about the little critics in your gut? Diversity and consistency. That means when they're hungry, they're not happy. And you may experience some irritating side effects, such as constipation, when your gut is not happy. To counteract this unpleasantness, add foods that are rich in probiotics to your diets, such as kefir, kombucha, or kraut. The Farmhouse Culture Gut Shots are great for any 500 calorie days, as every 1.5-ounce shot is full of live probiotics (10 billion CFUs) for only ten calories.

7. Berries

The added smoothie you want is loaded with supplements. Strawberries are a huge source of vitamin C, with a daily value of more than 100 percent in one cup. And that's not even the best part, a new study found that people who ate a flavonoid-rich diet, like those in blueberries and strawberries, had smaller rises in BMI over a 14-year period than those who didn't eat berries.

8. Eggs

One big egg contains six grams of protein and cooks in minutes. It is necessary to get as much protein as possible to keep your muscles full and build up. One study found people consuming an egg breakfast in place of a bagel were less hungry and ate less throughout the day. In other words, why not hard-boil some eggs when you are looking for something to do during your fasting period?

9. Nuts

They may be excessive in calories than many other snacks, but there is something in nuts that most junk foods don't have: good fat. Polyunsaturated fat in walnuts can indeed change the hunger and satiety physiological markers.

And if you think about calories, then don't be! A study conducted in 2012 showed that a one-ounce serving of almonds (about 23 nuts) had 20 percent fewer calories than those on the bottle. The chewing process essentially does not break down the almond cell walls entirely, leaving a part of the nut intact and unabsorbed during digestion.

10. Whole Grains

Being on a diet and eating carbs tend to belong to two different containers, but not always! Whole grains are rich in protein and fiber, so eating a little goes a long way to keep you full. Plus, a new study suggests consuming whole grains rather than refined grains could potentially revive your metabolism. So go ahead and eat all your grains, and try faro, bulgur, spelled, Kamet, amaranth, millet, sorghum, or freekeh out of your comfort zone.

11. Coffee

Technically, black coffee is a calorie-free drink, and a lot of people drink it with no adverse effects during fasting. There are some people who experience heart racing or stomach upset when using coffee during a strong, so track as you observe. You can have caffeinated or decaffeinated coffee, but there is a ban on any sweetener or milk. Spices such as cinnamon are absolutely fine!

Bonus:

Black coffee may, in fact, boost some of the benefits of intermittent fasting. This study showed that the ingestion of caffeine could support the production of the ketone. Coffee also has long-term proven to promote safe levels of blood sugar.

Go Easy on the Coffee

While black coffee is OK to drink while fasting intermittently, try not to go overboard. Too much coffee, especially if you are sensitive to caffeine, can leave you feeling jittery, anxious, and weak. Drinking coffee late in the day can affect your sleep quality too.

Besides, you're going to drink the coffee on an empty stomach, so the caffeine gets into your bloodstream quicker than if you'd just had a meal, and your stomach was full. Stick to a cup or two a day. If you want more, turn to decaf coffee.

12. Broths

For any time you decide to run for 24 hours or more, a bone or vegetable broth is recommended. Watch out for canned broths or cubes of bouillon, as these have loads of artificial flavors and preservatives that counteract the effects of your fast. The way to get there is an excellent homemade broth or one made from a trusted source.

13. Tea

Tea might just be the secret weapon that not only facilitates but also makes your fasting plan more successful. Of course, it help to increase your satiety!

All types of tea, including green, black, oolong, and herbal tea, are great to drink during a fast. But especially green tea has been shown to help increase satiety and promote healthy weight control. And tea usually improves the effectiveness of intermittent fasting by supporting gut health, probiotic balance, and cell safety.

14. Apple Cider Vinegar

Drinking apple cider vinegar has many health benefits, and you can definitely continue to drink it while fasting intermittently. And since apple cider vinegar helps support healthy blood sugar and digestion, the benefits of your intermittent fasting strategy may be enhanced.

Diluting a small quantity of apple cider vinegar in 8 ounces of water will not break your fast. Actually, it might be an excellent idea. Apple cider vinegar can lead to positive changes in metabolism that help to boost weight loss. Drinking apple cider vinegar daily can also reduce levels of total cholesterol, triglycerides, and LDL or "bad cholesterol."

However, make sure that you dilute it in water before you drink it. The acetic acid in apple cider vinegar is potent, and undiluted drinking may damage the enamel of the tooth.

Can You Avoid Drinks with Sugar?

Because of the large amount of sugar that Americans consume on average, most people have become dependent on glucose for energy rather than fatty acids. Each grocery store, pharmacy and coffee shop sells an array of sugary foods and drinks. Your body breaks it down and eventually stores it as body fat when you eat a lot of sugar, and sugar is not used for energy.

Additionally, the refined sugar found in most beverages quickly digests, spiking both your blood sugar and insulin levels. It is highly addictive too. The body just doesn't want more, and it needs more. Sugar and sweetened foods and beverages induce reward and craving reactions in the brain that are comparable to the responses triggered by addictive drugs that continue the cycle.

You drink sugary beverages, quickly digest them, and store the leftovers as body fat. You're experiencing a dramatic drop after the initial spike in blood sugar, which prompts you to eat more, and what happens? You are stocking up more fat. Because of this, it is best to avoid sugary drinks, such as soda, lemonade, fruit juices, sweetened iced tea, and even outright, whether or not you fast.

What about Soda Diet?

The diet soda contains no sugar, calories, or carbohydrates, so it may sound like it's OK for fasting, but it's not that easy. Diet soda and other soft beverages are filled with artificial sweeteners, which can lift sugar cravings dramatically, making fasting more difficult. Artificial sweeteners can also increase insulin resistance, making weight loss more difficult, and increasing your risk of developing diabetes.

People who drank sodas on diets tripled their belly fat over a nine-year period. The best way to avoid dietary soda and soft beverages entirely is to do so in moderation if you include them in your diet.

Weekly Diet Plan:

Here is the simple weekly diet plan for you, which helps you to makes you healthier and a recommendation for you. If you are doing intermittent fasting, you can plan your diet schedule according to this; this will help you to maintain the vitamin, protein level average in your body. You can manage the diet according to breakfast, lunch, and dinner.

Chapter 5: False Myths and Common Mistakes of Intermittent Fasting

Fasting is an ancient practice, but it is still an essential part of many cultures and religions that it is used today to bring spiritual clarity and mental focus. Fasting primarily for physical health is, however, a relatively new concept, and it spreads quickly because the results speak for themselves.

Intermittent fasting isn't complicated, but a lot of people just don't know what it is or the right way to do it. There has also come misinformation with the rising popularity of "IF" and a lack of specific training on how to follow a healthy intermittent fasting Strategy.

Do It! Intermittent Fasting Won't Reduce Your Metabolism!

False. This is our favorite bust myth because IF will increase your metabolism! Deprivation is never the target, and often this is a dangerous part of trying IF without the proper protocol and oversight. We also strongly encourage our customers to eat enough of the right macros (carbs, fats, and protein) to fuel their day properly and regulate hormones well. Every day, we simply eat at specific hours, rather than the whole day.

Several IF protocols exist which are safe and healthy. We practice the 16/8 etiquette at a faster way to fat loss. This ensures that during an 8-hour period, you can run for 16 hours out of your day and eat all of your daily meals. This may sound daunting, but bear in mind that for about half of your fast, you'll be asleep. The bodies should adapt and feel the benefits of daily rest and repair in just a couple of weeks or faster, versus continually digesting food.

We also suggest an occasional 24-hour fast to give the body extra healing and recovery time, but this should be prepared and requires specific nutrition "before and after." Also, we want to make sure that we use fasting as a health benefit rather than a strategy for starvation.

We still suggest the 16/8 protocol over either of these because, with 5/2 or alternating days, there is a much greater propensity to eat under.

Breakfast Is the Main Meal of the Day!

False. In fact, there is no research to back up this claim. You're only not going to find any scientific information that shows that eating first thing in the morning is essential–or even healthy. Breakfast food firms, which obviously have a significant financial stake in the game, have been heavily propagating the message. Skipping breakfast and eating more calories later in the day is a perfect way to extend the digestive rest of your body, so it can concentrate on recovery and repair.

Nevertheless, having the right foods is essential to break the fast later in the day (breakfast), which is a significant component of the faster way program.

Is There Anything I Can Eat or Drink During a Fasting Window?

Do not eat during the fasting period (which slows the rhythm and begins the digestive process), but you can drink non-sweetened, non-calorie beverages, including soda, black coffee, and tea. These will keep your body in digestive rest, and can also help push through the fasting window over the last few hours. Hydration is essential for the body to be able to repair itself and to flush out the toxins we bring every day!

Note: During their fast, some people use stevia to sweeten their coffee or tea, but the results may vary according to individuals. Watch the ingredients when using stevia powder. It's usually blended with other sweeteners. During your fast, do not use sugar, honey, maple syrup, or any kind of artificial sweetener.

Note also: If you enjoy "bulletproof" coffee (butter-and oil-mixed coffee), save this for your eating window. The high-fat content breaks your fast, and digestion begins.

When you usually eat every 3–4 hours and then suddenly shorten your eating time to an 8-hour period, you'll probably feel hungry and depressed all the time. Many people quit if they begin by fasting for too many hours without an adjustment period from a previous eating style. It takes 10 days to two weeks before you cease to feel hungry when you fast.

When a fast ends, it can be easy to overeat either because you feel ravenous or you justify to yourself that you are compensating for the lost calories. If you fast for weight loss and also because of other issues like stomach aches, this can backfire.

Most people are drinking water, black coffee, or tea whilst fasting. When you can't stand your coffee black, you may want to add a splash of milk or a sugar packet without realizing that these things break your tempo. Hold out your coffee butter and coconut oil.

It is also essential to avoid any protein-filled liquids, such as bone broth, because this can stop the cellular process that breaks down and recycles damaged molecules that you want to promote while fasting. You don't want anything heavily sweetened, though it's calorie-free. Zero-calorie sweeteners still have an adverse effect on insulin levels, which increases your appetite and makes you want to eat.

Intermittent fasting focuses on eating well, but largely overlooks food nutrient quality. Those who undergo intermittent fasting still need the same essential nutrients. In other words, if you stick to processed foods instead of whole grains, which consist of a well-balanced diet, intermittent fasting won't help you achieve your health goals.

If you've always had a pre-workout snack, it may seem foreign to practice while fasting. Yet, when there is no fuel, your body has plenty of energy stored in your body fat to use. As with any diet or exercise plan, checking with your doctor first is a good idea, but exercising with intermittent fasting can be safe.

Is This Safe to All?

Yes, intermittent fasting is good for everyone, but before you start practicing IF we always recommend a visit with your doctor. We don't recommend IF to kids, but people of all races, genders, ages, and backgrounds can practice intermittent fasting with safety. We warn you not to try IF on your own, though.

Alternatively, find a curriculum that you can trust to show you how to execute IF, and give you regular support and encouragement while you learn. It does not take long to learn, in truth. The faster way program, for example, is six weeks long, and most people have mastered the component of intermittent fasting by or before the halfway mark.

What If I Am on Diabetes?

While there is some promising work on diabetes subjects that use specific fasting procedures, it is essential that you check with your care provider before introducing anything new. Make sure to talk to your doctor about the particular essence of diabetes and the drugs involved before you participate in any health program. We worked with a number of Type 2 Diabetes clients who had their physician weaned off their drugs because of the health benefits.

What if I Get Hypothyroidism or Fatigue with the Adrenals?

If you are treated for hypothyroidism or adrenal tiredness, ease into intermittent fasting is important. More likely, you'll want to use the 12/12 fasting protocol rather than the 24-hour fast. Stick to whole foods if you have hypothyroidism or adrenal fatigue, eliminate gluten and dairy, and be sure to consume enough complex carbohydrates. Be aware of the balance between stress and rest, concentrate on sleep, and get enough sunlight within two hours of sunrise to keep your condition improving. Rest is a high priority for our digestive systems, for our minds and for our families in a faster way to fat loss. Rest is an essential investment for the wellbeing.

What Are Some Common Mistakes in IF?

The most significant error that we see is people trying IF without a trained professional's guidance. Many people want to try it alone, which is understandable as it seems so simple. The problem is that if you go into hunger mode and your body may even experience the opposite results of what you are hoping for, for example, without the right training and experience, you can actually cause damage!

The common mistake people make when they start practicing intermittent fasting on their own is under-hydration during their feeding window. The last thing you want to experience on your health journey is damage to your metabolism, exacerbation of adrenal fatigue, or long-term elevated levels of cortisol (stress hormone). By learning from an expert, you can avoid those pitfalls by investing a little of your time and money in yourself. You'll probably be able to do it after a few weeks without an expert.

Do I Need to Fast During A 24-Hour or Full-Day Work-Out?

No, during a 24-hour fast, we suggest that you rest or participate in an intense recovery workout. Active recovery workouts can be a long walk, a swim, or perhaps a hike. We recommend regular rest for optimum recovery as we work out during our sporadic fasts!

Is Intermittent Fasting Having a Negative Effect on Female Hormones or Fertility?

The honest response to this is yes, and no; it depends on what kind of intermittent fasting you practice. IF adversely affect fertility rates. The likelihood of under-eating is considerable with an alternative day protocol. No doubt, this kind of limited caloric intake will have a negative impact on the levels of female hormones.

You Jump Too Easily into Erratic Fasts

Many diets fail because they're such a radical deviation from our usual, regular way of eating that they often feel untenable. If you're adamant about the fasting principle, continue with a 12/12 approach for beginners where you fast for 12 hours a day and eat within the 12-hour window. That's probably quite close to what you're used to doing anyway, and who knows, maybe it's the only (if anyway) sustainable way to go along.

You're Choosing the Wrong Plan for Your Lifestyle

Again, by signing up for something you know will cramp your style, don't set yourself up for misery. If you're a night owl, don't plan to kick off at 6 p.m. If you're a daily gym-goer who every morning Integra their WOD and aren't willing to sacrifice your everyday spin, don't choose a schedule that severely restricts calories a couple of days a week. If you want to stick to some habit, you have to do it.

During the Feeding Time, You Eat So Much

This one is the most popular trap we'd expect people to fall into with IF. If you've chosen a particularly restrictive diet that leaves you hungry for hours of the day, the moment the clock says "it's time to eat," you'll probably go overboard for a week. Restrictive diets often don't work because we tend to get so mentally (and physically) deprived that we go hog crazy and overeat in a fit of starvation when we encourage ourselves to eat them.

During the Eating Window, You Don't Eat Enough

Yep, not eating enough is also a legitimate cause of weight gain, and we'll tell you why. Not eating enough cannibalizes your muscle mass, causing your metabolism to slow down while setting yourself up for a rebound similar to what we discussed with the last famous IF mistake. Without that metabolic muscle mass, you may be sabotaging your future ability to keep (never mind losing) fat. The challenge with IF is that since you eat according to some arbitrary temporal rules, rather than listening to the innate hints of your body, it's tough to know your real needs. If you are keen on doing the diet, be sure to talk to a registered dietitian to help you safely assess and meet your nutrient needs.

You Ignore What's in Favor of When

IF being a time-centered diet, most of the "plans" don't give any explicit rules about the types of food to eat during your "eating window," but that's not an excuse to stay on a French fries, milkshakes and beer diet. The fasts are not magic. Besides some small metabolic advantages, its primary impact on weight loss (if it even has one) is primarily based on the fact that you are limiting your number of eating hours and thus reducing the calorie consumption opportunities.

Unfortunately, if you choose the wrong kind of foods, the effect can be easily reversed. To get in the most nutrient-dense, nourishing foods during those days, change your focus from the idea of treating yourself during your restricting "feasting" hours. We recommend that every meal or snack is accompanied by a combination of satiating fiber, protein, and good fats to help carry you through your fasting.

Chapter 6: Which Are the Changes in Metabolism and Hormones in a Young Woman vs. Ageing Woman?

Hormones are broken down more slowly (metabolized) too. Many of the hormone-producing organs are also regulated by other hormones. Aging changes that process as well. An endocrine tissue, for example, can produce less of its hormone than it did at a younger age, or it can provide the same amount at a slower rate. When you change your diet, your hormones can also change; in this chapter, we define the frequent changes or effects of diet change due to fasting on your metabolism and hormones.

What are hormones, and how do they change?

The endocrine system is composed of hormone-producing organs and tissues. Hormones are naturally occurring chemicals formed in one location, released into the bloodstream, and then used by other target organs and systems.

Hormones control goal organs. Some organs have their own internal control systems, along with hormones, or instead.

When we age, the manner in which body systems are regulated naturally changes. Some target tissues become less responsive to their hormone, which controls them. The number of hormones released can change too.

Many hormones increase blood levels, many drops, and some remain unchanged. Hormones are broken down more slowly (metabolized) too.

Many of the hormone-producing organs are also regulated by other hormones. Aging changes the cycle as well. An endocrine tissue, for example, can produce less of its hormone than it did at a younger age, or it can provide the same amount at a slower rate.

Aging Changes:

In the brain is the hypothalamus. It produces hormones that control the other endocrine-system structures. The amount of these regulating hormones remains about the same, but the endocrine organ response may change as we age.

Also, within the brain is the pituitary gland. In the middle ages, this gland reaches its maximum size and then gradually becomes smaller. It has two parts:

- Hormones produced in the hypothalamus are stored in the back (post) part.

- The front (anterior) portion produces growth hormones, thyroid gland (TSH), adrenal cortex, ovaries, testes, and breasts.

In the neck lies the thyroid gland. It makes hormones that help control metabolism. The thyroid may get lumpy (nodular) with aging. With time, metabolism slows, starting at around the age of 20. Since thyroid hormones are developed and broken down at the same rate (metabolized), testing of the thyroid function is still carried out most regularly. The thyroid hormone levels may rise in some people, leading to an increased risk of death from cardiovascular disease.

The parathyroid glands are four tiny glands surrounding the thyroid. The parathyroid hormone affects the levels of calcium and phosphate, which affect the strength of the bone. The levels of the hormone parathyroid rise with age, which can lead to osteoporosis.

Insulin is produced through the pancreas. It lets sugar (glucose) migrate from the blood to the cells inside, where it can be used for energy.

The average level of fasting glucose increases from 6 to 14 milligrams per deciliter (mg) per 10 years after age 50, as the cells become less prone to insulin effects.

Over the kidneys lie the adrenal glands. The surface layer, the adrenal cortex, produces the aldosterone, cortisol hormones.

- Aldosterone regulates the balance of both fluids and electrolytes.

- Cortisol is the hormone called the "pain response." This stimulates glucose, protein, and fat breakdown, and it has anti-inflammatory and anti-allergic effects.

The release of aldosterone diminishes with age. This decrease may contribute to lightheadedness and a reduction in blood pressure with sudden changes of position (orthostatic hypotension). The release of cortisol also decreases with aging, but this hormone's blood level remains about the same. The levels of dehydroepiandrosterone also go down. The drop's effects on the body are not visible.

There are two functions to the ovaries and testes. They produce reproductive (ova and sperm) cells. They also provide the sex hormones which control the characteristics of secondary sex, such as breasts and facial hair.

- Men sometimes have lower testosterone levels with aging.

- After menopause, women have lower levels of estradiol and other hormones of the estrogen.

Effect of Changes:

Ultimately, some hormones are decreasing, some are not changing, and some are rising with age. Hormones generally decreasing include:

- Aldosterone

- Calcitonin

- Growth hormone

- Renin

In women, levels of estrogen and prolactin also decline dramatically.

The most commonly unchanged or only marginally reduced hormones include:

- Cortisol

- Epinephrine

- Insulin

- Thyroid hormones T3 and T4

6.1 Explaining the Effects of Fasting on Hormones

Hormone regulation (aka homeostasis) is so important to fulfill your dreams of health and wellness and make you feel good. Intermittent Fasting, combined with proper timing of nutrients, will help you achieve this hormone balance!

Used appropriately, intermittent fasting reverses insulin resistance, reduces chronic fatigue symptoms, normalizes menstrual cycles, and decreases anxiety.

Intermittent fasts are incredible, intestinal healing, and inflammation decreasing, hormone balancing tools that are used successfully with people ranging from professional athletes to IBS sufferers or chronic fatigue. Nevertheless, with this ancient healing technique growing in popularity, confusion has also increased. A common misconception is that intermittent fasting is just when you are not eating for a certain amount of time. This strategy would cause the body to become confused, have crazy spikes and drops in blood glucose levels, and eventually mess up the internal hormone balance that your body is trying to control so tightly. If you are interested in helping you reach your fitness goals, consider intermittent fasting.

So, What Are the Benefits of Regulating Hormones?

1. Diminished Insulin Resistance:

Insulin resistance is where the body cannot accept insulin (a glucose storage hormone) as much. It leads to Type 2 diabetes and disorders of fertility, including PCOS. Intermittent fasting has been found to increase your insulin sensitivity, which not only helps to reduce your risk of Type 2 Diabetes and PCOS, but also helps to tap into fat burning mechanisms that contribute to natural weight loss!

2. Increased Hormone Growth:

Growth hormone is needed to help your body burn fat and restore mass. And growth hormone levels are necessarily not measurable as soon as you eat. When you eat as soon as you wake up and snack until you go to bed, this does not encourage the growth hormone to get up and repair your muscles. On the other hand, intermittent fasting helps to increase the growth hormone by up to 2000 percent!

3. Diminished Cortisol + Increased Melatonin:

Specifically, a balance of cortisol (stress hormone) and melatonin (sleep hormone) occurs with appropriate nutrient timing combined with intermittent fasting. This is one of the most critical areas which is often overlooked when it comes to intermittent fasting. Melatonin is necessary to make you fall and stay asleep to feel relaxed and not groggy or exhausted the next day. In the morning, Cortisol is required to give you the energy and mental awareness to start your day.

This is one of the most common hormone imbalances I see, leading to weight gain, anxiety, poor sleep, and chronic tiredness. Incorporating proper timing of nutrients with intermittent fasting quickly helps you balance these essential hormones.

Hormone balance (aka homeostasis) is so important to fulfill your dreams of health and wellness and make you feel good. Intermittent fasting, combined with proper timing of nutrients, will help you achieve this hormone balance!

Effects on Hormones:

Here are few hormones and how it could affect them:

1. Hunger and hormones that store fat (ghrelin and leptin):

It's where intermittent fasting shines when it comes to improving the hormones that directly affect your appetite, blood sugar, and your metabolism. It has been shown that intermittent fasting reduces insulin resistance, which reduces the risk of diabetes and improves metabolism. It has also shown that intermittent fasting has a positive effect on the appetite hormone ghrelin. And, interestingly, the improvements in the release of ghrelin during IF increase brain dopamine levels, enhancing cognitive function (an example is a gut-brain axis at work in your body.)

If your blood sugar isn't steady, we recommend that you learn intermittent fasting procedures gradually, work softly with your body while you establish glucose control, and always talk to your doctor before making any dramatic lifestyle changes. Leptin resistance, another pattern of hormonal resistance which can lead to stubborn weight gain, was also shown to benefit from IF.

2. Female hormones (estrogen and progesterone):

The axis of the brain-ovary or of the hypothalamic-pituitary-gonadal (HPG) is the way the brain interacts with your ovaries. Your mind speaks to the ovaries by sending the hormones, which are simply chemical letters, and this causes your ovaries to release progesterone and estrogen. A healthy HPG axis is essential for your overall well-being and also for getting pregnant.

Women tend to be more prone to intermittent fasting, and this is partly due to something called kisspeptin. Women tend to have more kisspeptin, and research suggests that kisspeptin makes things like fasting more responsive. This can cause women wanting to skip their time of intermittent fasting, throw off their cycle, or just make them feel hormonally unbalanced overall. In theory, this could also affect both fertility and metabolism, but more studies need to be done.

Keep in mind that no two women are exactly the same. Clinically, we find some women with intermittent fasting do great, and some don't. Does that mean it shouldn't be done by women who are prone to intermittent fasting? Not quite. It may just take a more gentle approach to these individuals.

Here's precisely how to do fasting crescendo:

- Fast two nonconsecutive days a week (like Monday and Friday).

- Take it easy on food on fasting days. Light walking or gentle yoga, maybe.

- Fast shoot 12 to 16 hours.

- Try adding another day of fasting every two weeks (such as Tuesday, Thursday, and Friday).

- I typically suggest adding approximately 6 grams of branched-chain amino acid supplements (BCAAs) in powder and capsule form during this protocol. BCAAs help take the edge off and enhance the quick experience and positive impact.

3. Cortisol (Adrenal Hormones):

The primary stress hormone cortisol is secreted by the adrenal glands, which sit like little kidney caps on top of your kidneys. Adrenal fatigue is when the equilibrium between the brain and adrenal (HPA) is thrown out of whack. Cortisol will be high when low, low when high, or always high or low. For short, there are all kinds of dysfunctions of the HPA-axis. In general, though, many people found issues like this with circadian rhythm aren't rock stars with intermittent fasting. If you have a circadian rhythm dysfunction but still want to experiment with IF, start with a fasting crescendo or a protocol for beginners.

4. Thyroid hormones (T3 and T4):

Thyroid hormones affect each cell in your body, so be relaxed if your thyroid does not function well. Additionally, there are a lot of reasons a person can develop a thyroid hormone problem during his lifetime. For example, there are autoimmune thyroid problems such as Hashimoto's, thyroid conversion such problems as low T3 syndrome, thyroid resistance (similar to insulin resistance), and thyroid problems secondary to axis dysfunction of the brain-thyroid (HPT). Each of these thyroid hormone pathway disorders can respond to intermittent fasting differently, so treat it on a case-by-case basis and suggest consulting with a specialist in functional medicine.

6.2 Recommendations:

Doctors don't really know at this point whether the physiological decrease in raging hormones is average and healthy, or whether it should be treated. With a variety of ongoing large-scale experiments underway, new data are emerging all the time on whether and how hormones can be replaced.

Meanwhile, talking to your primary care doctor about treating any symptoms you experience is essential, and just as essential to prevent or manage symptoms by taking good care of yourself. If you do the intermittent fasting and if you're one of the millions of people suspecting they're having a hormone imbalance but don't know for sure, check out this guide to get more answers. If all of you are cleared to begin intermittent fasting, how do you start? Here are some suggestions:

One of the reasons why I personally think intermittent fasting has really taken over is because it is so easy to start. Literally, the only thing you really should know before you start is which sort of intermittent fasting schedule you intend to follow. And it's essential to understand the different types of intermittent fasting before you make that decision. Those are explained in detail in chapter 2.

6.3 How It Impacts Your Brain and Body Health

1. Can It Mess with Moods?

You've ever been hungry, and you know that an empty enough stomach can give way to irritable and angry feelings. Thanks to intermittent fasting, spend enough hours without food, and it is very likely that your mood will start taking a noticeable shift.

That's because of falling blood sugar levels and "a spike in cortisol (stress hormone),[which happens] when people get too hungry," drops and subsequent spikes when blood sugar "feasting" can be particularly bad for those with diabetes because it can cause a lack of blood glucose regulation and can trigger diabetes medication and insulin needs. "There's also a hormone called neuropeptide Y that signals people becoming more aggressive when they're starving (going back to the times of caveman, when you've only had to eat when you're fighting or having dinner)."

2. It Could Make You Even More Anxious:

The more adrenaline you're pumping through your system, the more likely you're feeling stressed. There is some evidence [that] restricted dietary activity may raise the stress hormone cortisol, which can cause changes in food preferences and cravings and mood. High levels of cortisol have also been associated with increased fat storage, so if you're trying to lose weight, IF might possibly work against you.

3. It Can Make You Tired:

While a study found that intermittent fasting might potentially improve your nightly, other studies indicate that it is more likely to cause sleep problems. According to a study, fasts can reduce the amount of REM sleep (the super-deep restorative shut-eye) due to the rise in cortisol and insulin from the body while fasting. (Good news, though: you may actually eat your way to sleep better.)

Depending on which intermittent fasting method you prefer, you can stop eating hours before bed, which may be good because eating near the bed isn't great for your health, potentially causing weight gain, acid reflux, and unnecessary gas, and sleeping difficulties. But an empty, growling stomach will make it hard to score some shut-eye. And, let's face it, your overall mental health is dependent on enough sleep: the following day changes in sleep behavior, consistency, and length will lead to fatigue and affect your mood.

4. Loneliness:

When you can't eat for specific periods of time, this can affect social interactions with friends and family that involve food. So losing out on friend time can lead to feelings of depression.

Skipping out on social commitments due to diet restrictions is also a common symptom of anorexia, and those with anorexia report having fewer friends, social activities, and less social support, per the National Association of Eating Disorders.

5. For Some, It May Increase the Risk of Developing Disordered Eating:

Both Albers-Bowing and Hertz agree that the strict rules of intermittent fasting about when you can and can't eat might trigger someone who has a history of an eating disorder or might be at risk for one.

At its heart, anorexia is about imposing limits and rigid rules on feeding, avoiding hunger and plenitude, and raising doubts about food, all of which have the ability to be perpetuated and intensified by IF.

The food may also cause "fear of loss of control (with food)" and "overeating on non-restricted days. Both of which are signs of binge eating disorder. However, one study found that women who reduced their caloric intake by 70 percent for four days and then ate "regularly" for three for a total of four weeks had more eating-related thoughts, increased fear of loss of control, and a regular diet.

6. According to Research, It Can Affect Your Cognitive Ability:

Fasting for long periods of time can lead you to take more rash, more short-term decisions.

You also change the neurotransmitters which are accessible within the brain when you fast. "And avoiding foods that raise your serotonin level may also cause you to have less of this feel-good chemicals in your brain," which can make you more impulsive. Think while making food decisions.

7. Your Perception of Hunger May Change:

 In its very core, intermittent fasting is about maintaining mental control over hunger and ignoring your body's signs of hunger (which, by the way, is triggered by a hormone called ghrelin).

Recent research suggests IF can also lower appetite and, in turn, help with weight loss by decreasing the hunger hormone ghrelin. These increases in ghrelin caused by IF may also raise the levels of dopamine (pleasure hormone) in the brain.

But hunger is like your neighbor knocking at your front door loudly. If you try to ignore the signals, it's like putting your hands over your ears and saying, "I can't hear them; maybe if I wait they're going to go away." Hunger tends to knock harder, hoping you're going to answer. Signs of hunger will eventually stop hurting if you don't respond. This destroys the desire for a good relationship.

If it could be harmful to anybody's food relationship, but particularly risky to those with a history of eating disorder. This is because they run a higher risk of using the rules and restrictions as a means to enable and exacerbate their eating disorder.

Chapter 7: Benefits of Intermittent Fasting for a Woman Over 50

You might have learned of intermittent fasting, which includes manageable, alternating eating, and not eating times, called fasting. Evidence is pretty clear that intermittent fasting is effective in many respects, and for older adults, this can be especially true.

Here are five benefits of intermittent fasting, and how to do it:

1. Intermittent Fasting Starts Cellular Repair Processes in Your Body:

Cellular damage is equal to the course as we age, but it has been shown that fasting induces cellular repair processes in your body, improves hormone function, and even improves the function of disease-related genes and longevity.

2. Intermittent Fasting Encourages Weight Loss, Especially Belly Fat:

Belly fat is a visceral fat indicator that lies deep inside the abdominal cavity that covers the organs and contributes to the disease.

Losing belly fat is difficult, especially as we age, but intermittent fasting can lead to a loss of four to seven percent of your waist circumference, according to a recent literature review. A recent study found that overall weight loss of three to eight percent over three to 24 weeks can result from intermittent fasting.

3. Intermittent Fasting Reduces Inflammation and Oxidative Stress:

Inflammation and oxidative stress are significant contributors to the disease as we age, and they lead to the noticeable signs of aging.

In overweight adults, intermittent fasting reduces markers of oxidative stress and inflammation

A vast body of research indicates that intermittent fasting is good for the brain, stimulating the growth of new nerve cells, protecting against stroke-related brain damage, and increasing levels of a hormone called a neurotropic brain-derived factor.

A recent study found intermittent fasting either postponed Alzheimer's onset or reduced its severity. Many studies show that intermittent fasting may offer protection against neurodegenerative diseases such as Parkinson's, Huntington's, and others.

5. Intermittent Fasting Can Extend Your Life:

A number of recent studies have also found that intermittent fasting has extended the life span of the participant. One study found that every other day fasting rats lived longer than non-fasting rats by 83 percent. In addition, the aging rate in the fasting rats was slowed, and their body weight and growth rates were lowered.

7.1 Shred Fat (Without Dieting or Limiting the Foods You Can Eat)

The diet you eat can have a significant impact on your weight. Some foods help with weight loss, such as full-fat yogurt, coconut oil, and eggs. Other foods can make you gain weight, mainly processed and refined products. This allows you to limit your diet and increase fewer fats.

Here are 11 foods to be avoided when you try to lose weight:

1. French fries and potato chips:

Whole potatoes are healthy and filling, but they are not French fries and potato chips. They are very high in calories, and too many of them are eaten quickly. Consumption of French fries and potato chips has been linked to weight gain in observational studies.

One study also found that potato chips could lead to higher weight gain per serving compared to any other food. What's more, baked, roasted, or fried potatoes that contain substances called acrylamides which cause cancer. Hence eating simple, boiled potatoes is excellent.

2. Sugary drinks:

Sugar-sweetened beverages, like soda, are among the planet's most unhealthy foods. These are strongly associated with weight gain, and when ingested unnecessarily, can have devastating health effects. While sugary drinks contain a lot of calories, they are not processed by your brain like solid food. Calories of liquid sugar don't make you feel whole, so you won't eat less to make up for. Then you end up adding these calories to your daily intake. If you're serious about weight loss, consider absolutely giving up on sugary drinks.

3. White bread:

White bread is highly refined, often with lots of added sugar. It's high on the glycemic index and can spike blood sugar. One analysis of 9,267 people found that eating two slices (120 grams) of white bread per day was associated with an increased risk of weight gain and obesity by 40 percent.

Fortunately, there are a lot of healthy alternatives to traditional wheat pieces of bread. One is Ezekiel bread, possibly the healthiest bread on the market.

Remember, though, that all wheat bread have gluten in them. Other options include bread oopsie, cornbread, and bread with almond flour.

4. Candy bars:

Candy bars are very unhealthy. We pack a lot of added sugar into a small package, including oils and refined flour. Candy bars are calorie-heavy and nutrient-poor. An average-sized chocolate-covered candy bar can contain about 200–300 calories, and even more, it can be listed in extra-large bars.

You can find candy bars everywhere, sadly. These are even strategically placed in stores so that customers are tempted to purchase them impulsively. If you crave a snack, instead eat a piece of fruit or a handful of nuts.

5. Most fruit juices:

Most fruit juices you find in the supermarket have very little to do with whole grain. The fruit juices are highly processed and sugar-loaded. These can actually contain just as much sugar and calories, if not more, than soda. Also, fruit juice is usually fiber-free and does not require chewing.

This means that a glass of orange juice will not have the same effects as an orange on its fullness, making it easy to consume large quantities in a short time period. Stay away from fruit juice, and instead eat the whole fruit.

6. Pastries, cookies, and cakes:

Pastries, cookies, and cakes are filled with unsanitary products such as added sugar and refined flour. These may also contain artificial Tran's fats, which are particularly toxic and are associated with many diseases.

Pastries, cookies, and cakes aren't very satisfying, and after eating these high-calorie, low-nutrient foods, you are likely to get hungry very soon. If you are craving something sweet, instead reach for a piece of dark chocolate.

7. Many alcohol forms (especially beer):

Alcohol offers more calories than carbs and protein, or about 7 calories per gram. However, there's no clear evidence of alcohol and weight gain. Drinking alcohol in moderation seems to be beautiful, and is positively associated with weight gain reduction. In contrast, heavy drinking is linked to increased weight gain. It also matters what form of alcohol is. Beer can cause weight gain, but it can actually be beneficial to drink wine in moderation.

8. Ice Cream:

Ice cream is amazingly delicious but very unhealthy. It's high in calories, and sugar is filled in most forms. Every now and then, a small portion of ice cream is good, but the problem is that it is effortless to consume massive amounts in one sitting. Try using less sugar and healthy ingredients like full-fat yogurt and fruit to make your own ice cream. Serve a small portion of yourself, then cut the ice cream so that you don't end up overeating.

9. Pizza:

Pizza is fast food that is very popular. Nonetheless, it also happens that pizzas made commercially are very unhealthy. These are disproportionately high in calories and often contain unhealthy ingredients such as highly refined meat and processed meat.

If you want to savor a slice of pizza, consider using healthy ingredients to make one at home. Homemade pizza sauce is also safer, as variations in supermarkets will contain lots of sugar.

10. High-calorie coffee drinks:

Coffee contains several biologically active substances, mainly caffeine. These chemicals can, at least in the short term, boost your metabolism, and increase fat burning. Nevertheless, those positive effects outweigh the adverse effects of adding unhealthy ingredients like added cream and sugar.

In reality, high-calorie coffee drinks are no better than soda. They are loaded with empty calories, which can be equal to an entire meal.

If you like coffee, sticking to regular, black coffee is better when you try to lose weight. It's good to add a little cream or milk too. Only avoid adding sugar, creamers high in calories, and other unhealthy ingredients.

11. Foods rich in added sugar:

Perhaps the worst thing in the modern diet is added sugar. Excess levels have been related to some of today's world's most dangerous diseases. Foods high in added sugar usually have lots of empty calories, but they are not very full. Sugary breakfast cereals, granola bars, and low-fat, flavored yogurt are examples of foods that may contain massive amounts of added sugar.

While buying "low-fat" or "fat-free" foods, you should be especially careful, because manufacturers often add lots of sugar to compensate for the taste that is lost when the fat is taken away.

7.2 Increase Your Energy Levels

Go to the pharmacy, and you will see a multitude of vitamins, herbs, and other supplements believed to be boosters of energy. Some are even supplemented with soft drinks and other foods. But there is little or no scientific evidence that energy boosters such as ginseng, guarana, and picolinate chromium actually work. Fortunately, there is some work you can do to improve your own levels of natural energy:

1. Command Stress:

Stress-induced emotions consume enormous amounts of energy. Can it all help to spread tension by talking to a friend or family, attending a support group or seeing a psychotherapist? Relaxation techniques such as meditation, self-hypnosis, yoga, and tai chi are also useful tools for stress reduction.

2. Lighten Up Your Load

Overwork is one of the root causes of fatigue. Overwork can include social, family, and professional obligations. Consider streamlining your 'must-do' list of activities. Set the goals as to the most significant events. Pare down the less important ones. If need be, consider asking for additional help at work.

3. Exercise:

Exercise almost guarantees you will sleep better. It also gives your cells more burning energy, and oxygen circulates. So exercise causes the body to release epinephrine, so norepinephrine, stress hormones, which can make you feel energized is available in modest amounts. Even a brisk walk represents a good start.

4. Evicting Smoking

You realize smoking is a hazard to your safety. But you may not know that your energy is potentially siphoned off by smoking triggering insomnia. Tobacco nicotine is a stimulant, thereby accelerating heart rate, increasing blood pressure, and enhancing wakefulness-related brain-wave activity, making it easier to fall asleep. And once you fall asleep, with cravings, its addictive strength will kick you in and wake you up.

5. Restrict Your Sleep:

When you believe you may be deprived of sleep, try to sleep less. This advice may sound strange, but determining how much sleep you actually need can reduce the amount of time you spend not sleeping in bed. This makes it easy to fall asleep, and it encourages more restful sleep over the long term. How to do this:

• Stop daytime napping.

• Go to bed later than usual the first night, and just sleep for four hours.

• If you like you've been sleeping well during the four-hour period, add another 15–30 minutes of sleep the following night.

• As long as you sleep comfortably all the time you're in bed, keep adding rest gradually on the nights that follow.

6. Eat For Energy:

Eating small meals and snacks every few hours is better than eating three large meals a day. This strategy will reduce your fatigue perception because your brain needs a constant nutrient supply.

Eating foods with a low glycemic index whose sugars are absorbed gradually will help you avoid energy loss, usually occurring after consuming fast-absorbed sugars or refined starches. Low glycemic index foods include whole grains, high-fiber vegetables, nuts, and healthy oils like olive oil. High-carbohydrate diets are generally given the highest glycemic index. Proteins and fats have strictly zero glycemic indexes.

7. Using Caffeine to Your Advantage:

Caffeine helps to increase alertness, and having a cup of coffee may help to make the mind clearer. But if you want to get the energizing effects of caffeine, you need to use it carefully. It can cause insomnia, especially if eaten in large quantities or after 2 p.m.

8. Restrict Alcohol:

One of the strongest hedges against the midnight drop is not to drink alcohol at lunchtime. Especially at midday, the sedative effect of alcohol is high. Similarly, avoid a cocktail at five o'clock, if you want to have energy for the evening. If you are going to drink, at a time when you don't mind having your energy wind down, do so in moderation.

9. Drink Water:

What's the only nutrient shown to improve performance for all but the most demanding endurance activity? It is not a precious drink of sports. That is wind. One of the first symptoms, if your body is deprived of fluids, is a sense of exhaustion.

7.3 Heighten Your Testosterone and Growth Hormone Production

Human growth hormone (HGH) is an essential hormone which your pituitary gland produces.

Also named as growth hormone (GH), it plays a crucial role in development, cell repair, body composition, and metabolism. HGH also boosts muscle growth, strength, and performance in exercise while helping you recover from injury and illness.

Low levels of HGH can lower your quality of life, increase your risk of illness, and make you gain fat. Especially during weight loss, injury recovery, and athletic training, optimal rates are significant. Interestingly, choices about your diet and lifestyle can have a substantial effect on your HGH levels.

Here are evidence-based approaches to naturally raise levels of the human growth hormone (HGH):

1. Lose Body Fat:

The volume of belly fat that you are carrying is directly related to the output of your HGH. Those with higher levels of abdominal fat are likely to have decreased development of HGH and increased risk of illness.

One study found that those with three times the amount of belly fat as the control group had less than half the amount of HGH that they had. Another research tracked the release of HGH lasting 24 hours and found a significant decrease in those with more abdominal fat. Ironically, research suggests excess body fat has a more significant effect on men's HGH levels. Lowering body fat remains essential for both genders, however.

Furthermore, a study found that humans with obesity had lower levels of HGH and IGF-1, a protein associated with development. After a substantial weight loss, their rates returned to normal.

Belly fat is the most harmful type of fat stored and is associated with many diseases. Losing belly fat can help optimize the HGH rates as well as other safety aspects.

2. Intermittently Fast:

Studies show that fasting leads to higher rates of HGH. One study found that HGH rates rose by more than 300 percent for 3 days. They had been increased by a vast 1.250 percent after 1 week of fasting. Other studies have found similar effects after just 2–3 days of fasting, with double or triple levels of HGH. Continuous fasting, however, is not sustainable over the long term. Intermittent fasting is a more common dietary method, limiting eating to short periods of time.

There are several strategies for intermittent fasting. One common approach is a daily eating window of 8 hours with a fast of 16 hours. This includes eating only 500–600 calories 2 days a week.

Intermittent fasting can help in two main ways to optimize the HGH levels. First, it can help you to drop body fat, which has a direct effect on the production of HGH.

Second, since insulin is released when you eat, it will keep your insulin levels down for most of the day. Research suggests your natural growth hormone may be disrupted by insulin spikes.

One research found significant differences in fasting-day HGH levels compared to eating-day. It is also possible that shorter 12–16-hour fasts would benefit, though more research is needed to compare their effects with full-day fasts.

3. Consider an Arginine Supplement:

Arginine will boost HGH if taken alone. Although most people use amino acids such as arginine alongside exercise, there are several studies that show little or no increase in HGH levels.

Studies have, however, observed that taking arginine alone without any exercise significantly increases these hormone levels. Other non-exercise studies also support arginine utilization to boost HGH.

One study shows the effects of taking either 45 or 114 mg arginine per pound of body weight (100 or 250 mg per kg) or about 6–10 or 15–20 grams per day, respectively.

This found no effect on the lower dose, but participants taking the higher dose experienced an increase in HGH levels about 60 percent during sleep.

4. Reduce Your Sugar Intake:

 Lower HGH levels are associated with an increase in insulin content. Refined carbs and sugar mostly raise levels of insulin, so reducing your intake can help optimize growth hormone. One study found that healthy people had HGH levels 3–4 times higher than those with diabetes, and reduced carb tolerance and insulin control.

In addition to directly affecting levels of insulin, excess sugar consumption is a critical factor in weight gain and obesity, which also affects levels of HGH. That said, the occasional sweet treat won't have a long-term effect on your HGH rates. Look for a balanced diet, since what you eat has a profound effect on your health, hormones, and structure of your body.

5. Do Not Eat Much Before Bedtime:

Your body releases substantial amounts of HGH naturally, especially at night. Because most of the meals cause insulin levels to rise, some experts suggest avoiding food before bedtime.

A high-carb or high-protein meal, in particular, can spike up your insulin and potentially block some of the HGH released at night. Keep in mind that there is not enough work on this theory. Nonetheless, insulin levels usually decrease 2–3 hours after eating, so you might want to avoid meals dependent on the carb or protein 2–3 hours before bedtime.

6. Take a GABA Supplement:

Gamma-aminobutyric acid (GABA) is named as the non-protein amino acid that functions as a neurotransmitter and sends out signals around your brain. It is often used to help sleep, as a well-known soothing agent for your mind and central nervous system. It may also help to increase your HGH levels, interestingly. One research found that taking a GABA supplement led to an increase in HGH at the rest of 400 percent and an increase of 200 percent after exercise. GABA can also raise levels of HGH by enhancing your sleep, as the release of your growth hormone at night is related to sleep quality and profundity.

Most of these improvements, however, have been short-lived, and the long-term benefits of GABA for growth hormone levels remain unclear.

7. High-Intensity Exercise

Exercise is a successful way to raise HGH rates dramatically. The change depends on the type of exercise, speed, food intake around the workout, and the proper characteristics of your body. High-intensity exercise raises HGH the most, but it helps all forms of exercise.

In order to spike your HGH levels and maximize fat loss, you can perform repeated sprints, interval training, weight training, or circuit training. Including vitamins, exercise is primarily responsible for short-term increases in HGH rates.

Nevertheless, exercise will improve your hormone activity over the long term, and decrease body fat, both of which support your HGH levels.

8. Take Beta-Alanine and/or a Sports Drink During Your Workouts:

Many sports supplements may improve output and raise your HGH levels temporarily. For one test, taking 4.8 grams of beta-alanine before a workout increased, by 22 percent, the number of repetitions done. It also doubled peak power and increased levels of HGH relative to the non-supplement community.

Another research has shown that a sugary sports drink has increased levels of HGH towards the end of a workout. If you try to lose fat, however, the extra calories of the drink will negate any benefit from the spike of short-term HGH.

Studies have shown that protein shakes can boost HGH levels around workouts, both with and without carbs. Nevertheless, if a casein or whey protein supplement is taken immediately before exercising energy, the opposite effect may be that.

One research found that drinking a 25 gram (0.9 ounces) casein or whey protein drink 30 minutes before strength exercise decreased human growth hormone and testosterone levels compared to a non-caloric placebo.

9.　**Optimize Your Sleep**:

Some HGH is released in bursts when you're sleeping. Such pulses are based on the inner clock or circadian rhythm of your body. Before midnight, the highest pulses occur, with some smaller pulses in the early morning. Research has shown that poor sleep can reduce the body's amount of HGH. Yes, having an adequate amount of deep sleep is one of the best strategies to improve the HGH output over the long term.

10. Take Melatonin Supplement:

Melatonin is a hormone that plays a vital role in regulating sleep and blood pressure. Melatonin supplements are becoming a popular sleep aid that can improve the quality and duration of your sleep.

Although good sleep alone can support levels of HGH, further work has shown that a melatonin supplement can directly increase the development of HGH. Melatonin is pretty safe and non-toxic too. Nonetheless, it may, in specific ways, change your brain chemistry, so you may want to consult with your healthcare provider before you use it.

Take 1–5 mg about 30 minutes before going to bed, to optimize its effectiveness. Start by taking a lower dose to assess your tolerance and then increase if necessary.

11. Try these additional natural supplements:

Several other supplements may increase the production of human growth hormones, including:

- Glutamine: A dose of 2 grams will temporarily increase levels to 78%.

- Creatine: A 20-gram dose of creatine raised HGH levels dramatically for 2–6 hours.

- Ornithine: One research gave ornithine to participants 30 minutes after exercise, and observed a higher peak in HGH rates.

- Dopa: L. 500 mg of L-dopa increased HGH levels for up to 2 hours in patients with Parkinson's disease.

- Glycine: Studies have found that glycine is capable of improving exercise efficiency and producing short-term HGH spikes.

While these supplements can increase your levels of HGH, studies show that their effects are temporary only.

7.4 Improve Your Cognitive Functioning

We usually associate the term "cognitive development" with children and infants. While many adults do not think about cognitive development, they should do so, especially since studies show that reduced cognitive function can prematurely age us and lower life expectancy. In the medical community, it is well known that people who have advanced stages of Alzheimer's or dementia don't live as long as those who are free of these conditions.

By making confident lifestyle choices, including those that tax or challenge the brain, you can be many years younger than your chronological age. Research-wise, the past 20 years have shown that new neurons and new synapses can be generated by some areas of the adult brain. (For example, here's one recent study.) Mostly, whenever we learn something new, engage in new activities, or even think about a new concept, the brain will rewire itself in response to these activities. As with babies, adults can continue to grow their minds and protect cognitive functioning as they age.

There are many positive ways of building better memory and reducing the chances of developing diminished cognitive ability, dementia, or later Alzheimer's in life, all of which make us act old and feel old.

Here are ten of them:

1. Exercise to Improve the Cognitive Function:

Exercise increases blood flow to the hippocampus, which is the memory part of the brain. A recent study found that in those who were aerobically fit, the loss of tissue density in mind was less, which is another way of saying fit people have better cognitive functioning. Many other studies show that exercise improves one's ability to learn, manage stressful situations, make clear choices, and remember memories and information.

2. Watch TV and Read "Actively."

How active your brain has to be is the difference between watching *The Bachelorette* and watching an educational science show. Watching television is cognitively enriching when it takes an effort to understand what you are watching or when it sparks questions, ideas, or moments of "aha." As for reading, the same is true. It takes less brain power to flip through a celebrity tabloid magazine than, say, a magazine such as Smithsonian. Build new connections within your brain by reading something that is instructive rather than just entertaining. Make yourself recall what you've just learned after reading or watching TV. The training increases retention.

3. Take Up a New Hobby:

Enhance cognitive stimulation through embarking on a new active activity involving thinking, as compared to just attending a baseball game or concert. Some examples include: gardening, antiquing, taking in an instrument, raising chickens, learning a foreign language, or selling items on the Internet. Read books, talk with experts, take classes, attend conferences, or join hobby-related organizations. All of this learning activity develops new neuronal connections, helping to offset cell loss due to aging or illness.

4. Solve All Sorts of Puzzles:

Puzzles are a great way to build new connections within the brain. There are many different types of puzzles, including crosswords. Among these are the acrostics, cryptograms, and many other word-oriented brains teasers. Many brain teasers are total without words like Sudoku. Seeking a variety is particularly good for your brain. Or start with one type, and then move to another type of puzzle as you get stronger. With each particular type of puzzle, your brain will be challenged once more. Switching from a simple puzzle to a more challenging or unfamiliar form induces new brain activity, or learning since your brain now has to generate new memories to master the new challenge.

5. Play Board Games and Card Games:

Games involving strategy are excellent for the brain, especially those involving puzzle solving or some kind of new learning, such as Scrabble, Wheel of Fortune, Jeopardy, Trivial Pursuit, Monopoly, and Who Wants to Be a Millionaire, all available in digital form. Chess and checkers are great games because almost every game is unique, and a different set of strategies is needed each time. Card games can help preserve cognitive functioning equally because the player tries to refine the most effective strategies according to the play style of the opponent. You can use a computer to play card games too!

6. Visit Museums, Zoos, and Historical Sites:

There are plenty of specialized museums as well as zoos and historical sites that will help you build a better understanding. Don't be a passive visitor to get the most out of the visit from a cognitive standpoint. Read the signs next to the displays, try to repeat the key information to yourself, then do it once or twice during or after your stay. Not only will you understand what the shows were about, but also you'll increase the odds of being able to remember the details months or even years later with some sporadic recall attempts.

7. Become a Student Again:

A number of continuing education classes are available that don't allow you to be in a degree program that you just sign up for when you feel like it. Relatively cheap courses are offered by community colleges. As a student, you will have many chances of learning new things, and most teachers will give you assessments that will force you to recall the learned knowledge. In many places, no-degree classes are offered, from technical subjects to local community history, public speaking, relationships, art, and other fun subjects.

8. Attend Workshops:

Workshops, conferences, and other gatherings where experts in their field share their knowledge offer a different way of building cognitive function through active learning. While these are usually offered in the career of an individual, several others may be found connected to hobbies and personal interests. For starters, one that recently came across my desk has been a workshop on how to trace the origins of your family. Another was astronomy for the amateur backyard.

9. Cut Back On Work:

People with high-stress levels are more likely to suffer from cognitive problems than those who are stress-free. Although medicines can relieve stress symptoms, they don't cure the problem or help you understand the root cause of the stress that's important. Since many medications need ever-increasing dosages to be successful, and many have side effects, it is important to consider reducing stress in more natural ways, including exercise, naps, individual counseling, meditation, calming activities, spiritual growth, and other means.

10. Address Depression:

Depressed individuals are more likely to suffer later in life from cognitive problems than those free from depression. As with stress, many depressed people simply run to their family doctor and say, "Can you give me something to be depressed?" And with a prescription, go away. No attempt is made to figure out, let alone cure, what triggers the depression in the first place. As with stress, besides treatment, there are ways to deliver a long-lasting solution to depression, including individual counseling, exercise, spiritual growth, career rejuvenation, goal setting, and other strategies.

Chapter 8: Intermittent Fasting and Autophagy

Intermittent fasting isn't just a technique for weight loss or a trick that bodybuilders use to lose fat while retaining lean muscle mass quickly. It is a healthy lifestyle told by human evolution and metabolism research to its best. This asks the human body to be far more powerful and self-protective than it is used to in modern times.

The 5 stages of intermittent fasts with the LIFE Fasting Tracker app:

1) Ketosis and substantial ketosis,

2) Autophagy,

3) Growth hormone,

4) Insulin reduction,

5) Rejuvenation of immune cells

The individual cell within your body is in "development" mode in a well-fed environment. The insulin signaling and motor pathways are active and tell the cell to expand, divide, and synthesize proteins. Such channels, by the way, have effects on cancer growth when they are overactive.

The "kanamycin mammalian target" or mTOR loves to have abundant nutrients around it, particularly carbohydrates and proteins. Once involved, mTOR tells the cell not to bother with autophagy (literally cellular "self-eating"), a cycle of recycling and washing, ridding the body, for example, of degraded and misfolded proteins. The well-fed cell is not worried about being productive, and recycling its components-growing and dividing is too busy.

The cells and their elements are heavily acetylated in a well-fed environment too. This means that different molecules in your cells are "decorated" with acetyl groups on their lysine (amino acid) residues, including the "packaging" proteins called histones that wrap your DNA up nicely within the core of your cells. Don't worry if the last paragraph indicates you don't understand the jargon. What you really have to know is that the well-fed cell switches on a lot of genes, including those linked to cell survival and proliferation. This is because acetylation loosens the proteins in the packaging that usually keep your DNA wrapped in and allow you to read your protein DNA.

When your cells turn on the genes of cell growth and proliferation when you're not fasting, they turn off other genes too. These include fat metabolism-related genes, stress tolerance, and repair damage. When you fast, some of your fat becomes ketone bodies that appear to reactivate these genes, resulting, for example, in lowering inflammation and stress resistance in the brain.

But things are very different during starvation. When you are hard, your body reacts to what it sees as a stress on the environment (low food availability) by modifying the expression of genes that are important to protect you from stress, well.

We have a well-preserved "system" for the starvation that pushes our cell into an entirely different state when food, mainly glucose or sugar, is not around. You activate the AMPK signaling route while fasting, and when exercising. AMPK or AMP-activated protein kinase 5' is the brake on the gas pedal of mTOR. AMPK points the cell into the self-protective mode, activating autophagy, and breakdown of fat. It does inhibit mTOR. While you're fasting at the same time, the levels of a molecule called NAD+ start to rise because you don't have the dietary proteins and sugars around which the Krebs cycle normally converts NAD+ into NADH.

NAD+ stimulates the sirtuins, SIRT1 and SIRT3, a receptor whose counterpart is vitamin B3. (Have you heard of the "long-life" molecule called resveratrol in wine? Yes, it became famous as a possible sirtuin activator). These sirtuins are proteins that remove from histones and other proteins the acetyl groups we spoke about above. In this process, the sirtuins silence cell-proliferation genes and activate proteins involved in creating new mitochondria (your cells ' power-generating factories) and cleaning up reactive oxygen species.

Ketones also produced during fasting, work as inhibitors of deacetylase (i.e., maintaining acetyl groups). It flips on antioxidant-related genes and damage repair processes.

Whew, that's happening a lot while your body doesn't take any calories. But when are these things happening exactly? We've helped you to visualize the timeline below and in the LIFE Fasting Tracker app, with a series of icons on the LIFE fasting arc representing the five fasting stages!

The Five Stages of Fasting Intermittent (and Prolonged)

1. You reached the metabolic condition called ketosis by 12 hours. Your body begins to break down in this state, and burn fat.

The liver uses some of that fat to create ketone bodies. When glucose is not readily available, ketone bodies, or ketones, serve as an alternative energy source for your brain cells and cells in other tissues. Did you know that when your body is in a resting state, your brain uses about 60 percent of your glucose? When you're fasting, your liver-generated ketone bodies partially substitute glucose as a fuel for your brain and other organs. This use of ketone by your brain is one of the reasons why fasting is often believed to encourage mental clarity, and positive mood – ketones generate fewer inflammatory products as they are metabolized than glucose, and they can even kick-start BDNF growth factor output!

2. You moved to the fat-burning mode by 18 hours, and generate significant ketones. Now you can start measuring blood ketone levels above the baseline values (such as around a range of 0.6 to 1.0).

When your bloodstream levels rise, ketones may serve as hormones - like signaling molecules to tell the body, for example, to ramp up stress-busting pathways that minimize inflammation and repair damaged DNA.

Your cells are increasingly recycling old components within 24 hours and breaking down misfolded proteins linked to Alzheimer's disease and other diseases. This process is known as autophagy.

If your cells are unable to start autophagy, then bad things happen, like neurodegenerative diseases. Autophagy is an essential process in the rejuvenation of cells and tissues – it eliminates damaged cellular components, including misfolded proteins. Fasting activates the signaling path of the AMPK and inhibits mTOR activity, which enables autophagy in turn. However, this only begins to happen naturally when your glucose stores are substantially depleted, and your insulin levels begin to drop.

3. After 48 hours without calories, or with very little calories, carbohydrates, or proteins, the growth hormone level is up to five times higher than when fasting began.

A portion of the reason for this is that the ketone bodies produced during fasting, for example, in the brain, promote growth hormone secretion. The appetite hormone, Ghrelin, also stimulates the release of growth hormones. The growth hormone helps preserve lean muscle mass and lowers the accumulation of fat tissue, especially as we age. It appeared to play a role in the longevity of mammals, and may promote cardiovascular and wound healing.

4. Your insulin has fallen to its lowest point by 54 hours since you started fasting, and your body is becoming increasingly insulin-sensitive.

Lowering your insulin levels offers a range of health benefits both in short and the long run. Higher insulin levels put a brake on the signaling pathways for insulin and mTOR, and activate autophagy. Lower insulin levels can reduce inflammation, make you more sensitive to insulin (and/or less resistant to insulin, which is especially useful if you have a high risk of developing diabetes), and protect you from chronic aging diseases, including cancer.

5. Your body breaks down old immune cells by 72 hours and generates new ones.

Prolonged fasting reduces circulating levels of IGF-1 and PKA activity in different populations of cells. IGF-1, or insulin-like growth factor 1, looks very much like insulin and has growth-promoting effects on almost every body cell. IGF-1 activates signaling pathways that promote cell survival and growth, including the PI3K-Akt trail. Also, PKA can activate the mTOR pathway (and, interestingly, too much caffeine can encourage PKA activation during a fast).

You can see where this leads–by putting the brakes on IGF-1 and PKA by nutrient restriction and fasting, cell survival pathways can be turned down, and old cells and protein breakdown and recycling. Studies in mice have shown that extended fasting (greater than 48 hours) leads to stress tolerance, self-renewal and regeneration of hematopoietic or blood cell stem cells by growing IGF-1 and PKA. Through this same mechanism, prolonged 72-hour fasting in patients undergoing chemotherapy has been shown to preserve healthy white blood cells or lymphocyte counts.

Chapter 9: Suggestions for a Woman Over 50

As the years go by, many women find that, in their 40s and 50s, the lifestyle that worked in their 20s and 30s fails to achieve the same results. When women enter their 50s (the average age of menopause onset), they will have to make up for changes in hormonal, cardiovascular, and muscle rates.

For aged women, weight gain is average due to reductions for muscle mass, accumulation of excess fat, and a lower metabolic rate of rest. Hormonal shifts can cause a lot of symptoms and increase the overall risk of heart and stroke disorders. And specific nutrient absorption can decrease as a result of a loss of stomach acid. So many women want to lose weight and are interested in intermittent fasting. There are tips in this complete guide that you can follow your fasting routine.

9.1 How to Track Progress While Fasting

Intermittent fasting requires commitment, strict scheduling, and a great deal of resistance to temptation. That is to say, it is not the most straightforward diet out there. To make things even more tricky, once you decide to try it out, you still have to determine what kind of fasting you'll do: alternate-day fasting,

16:8 diet (where you fast for 16 hours and eat in an 8-hour window), 5:2 food (where you usually eat five days a week and eat very fewer calories two days a week), eat-stop-eat, Warrior diet, the list goes on.

Does it all sound complicated kind of? Yes. But thankfully, your smartphone or tablet will make it as simple as it is for you, so you'll hardly even have to think about whether or not it's time to eat. There is no lack of intermittent fasting software designed to help you monitor your fasting hours and keep you on schedule, as well as keeping tabs on your weight changes with graphs and journaling. The only tricky part is to find out which device is your fava.

When you're looking for an intermittent fasting program app, first consider what your objectives are. Would you like the app to track your fasting time? Is it monitoring your progress? Or helping with planning the meals? It's time to look at what's out there once you've learned what you want an app to do to you.

Here are intermittent fasting apps approved by dietitians designed to make it easier to follow any type of IF plan:

1. If You Want a Quick Reminder While Eating: Zero:

Zero can be configured to track your fasting hours, which means it works no matter what type of IF program you're on (even if you've made up your own schedule). You can choose from several pre-set fasting times, or build your own plan for up to seven days.

The design is clean and straightforward, with a dashboard that can help you evaluate your fasting patterns over time, making it easy to navigate.

2. If You Want to Keep Track of Your Fasting Times and Control Your Diet: Fasten

Fasten is one of the more detailed monitoring software out there, enabling you to keep track of your food intake and keep track of your overall progress. It has a broad, accessible interface that leaves plenty of space for journaling, displaying your data in easy-to-read graphs, and accessing your device or desktop information.

3. If You Want Advice About Meal-Planning: Body Fast:

Remember when we said that there were a lot of different fasting plans? Well, Body Fast gives you 10 different choices and loads of tips for coaching and meal planning too. If you're committed to IF but are struggling with its day-to-day mechanics, this app could give you what you need to solve your problems.

The Body Fast coach gives tips based on data such as your age and weight loss goals, but this is not a substitute for working with a medical professional like a registered dietitian who can genuinely customize your meal plan to suit your own unique needs.

4. If You Like Community Support: Vora:

This is a standard IF tracking app (providing fasting/goal timing and progress on weight loss). But it does include one unique and essential component: support for the community.

Evidence has shown that transparency and social support contribute to more progress in behavioral change. By engaging in a community of like-minded people, this app can help you keep up with your IF plan for the best results over the long term.

So if one of your friends is doing IF and you need peer-to-peer motivation, Vora may be the perfect fit for that.

5. If You Want To Test Different Fasting Plans: Fast Habit:

If you change your fasting goals all the time (like doing 5:2 a week and alternating days fasting the next), then Fast Habit is one of the best ways to keep up with your schedule. Simply set up the required fasting window in the app when you're ready to go and start. This synchronizes on - the-spot transparency and comprehensive health monitoring with Apple Watch and Apple Fitness.

You can also set up notifications and remainder for yourself, or through the simple dashboard check your fasting stats over the last 10 days, but tracking more than that will require a premium membership.

6.   **If You Are on The Keto Diet As Well: LIFE Fasting Tracker**:

LIFE Fasting Tracker works for IF schedule tracking, as it allows you to set the start and end times and goals for the duration of your fasting periods. This app can help you track how long you've actually been in ketosis if you're focused on a keto diet. You can also communicate with friends using the app to fast together and help motivate one another.

7. If You Like Accountability for Social Media: Ate Food Diary:

The Ate Food Diary enables you to keep a visual food diary, keep track of how much time has passed between meals and snacks, and provide a simple way to look back on the food choices you made and how they made you feel. If you are in accountability for social media, Ate makes it easy to share what you've eaten on your channels.

Chapter 10: Exercises that Can Help to Lose Weight After 50

To understand the science of intermittent fasting, the basics of nutrition need to be looked into. And it's pretty straightforward: the food we eat is broken down into molecules and ends up in our blood that feeds our bodies' cells. Net carbohydrates (all carbs in the meal minus the fiber) are part of those molecules, and our body turns them into sugar (glucose), so our cells could use them for energy. To be able to use sugar for power, we need insulin, which is produced in our pancreas every time we throw carbohydrates into some food.

Any excess sugar we don't eat gets stored in the form of fat with the expectation that we'll use that fat for energy later, once we've got no sugar left. The right way to NOT end up with vast stores of fat (and become overweight) is to spend the same amount of energy you get from the food. Life, however, isn't perfect, and many of us have habits that restrict our chances of moving all day long. As a matter of fact, office workers tend to sit 75 percent of their waking hours. So, what should we do to lose weight or not gain weight?

One way to do this is to focus on increasing your energy consumption by increasing physical activity or in terms of a layman–exercising and doing sport. But you already knew that one, right? Another approach, though, is to concentrate on consuming less food than you need for the energy that day, generating a caloric deficit as a result. And this is where intermittent fasting enters.

Intermittent fasting facilitates the reduction of the number of meals and calories you eat per day. For some time, it is much more convenient not to eat at all vs. eating less Restricting meal frequency ends up reducing insulin to low enough levels and long enough to get our bodies into ketosis mode–a magical state where we use fat for energy vs. sugar. And as a result, you are losing weight. But please be careful-it will only be beneficial to reduce the number of meals or the number of hours you eat per day if you consume fewer calories than you need.

The good news, right? You can altogether avoid metabolic syndrome, and "it's never too late to start exercising," we have middle-aged people going to the gym who have never worked out and rowing a half-marathon within four months. Exercising is even more successful when paired with a healthy diet. There are some obstacles to get your exercise groove on after age 50: women experience age-related declines.

1. Walking:

Not only is it a great way to lose weight because you don't need to be part of a gym or invest in special equipment, but it's also a perfect workout for older adults because it's gentle on your joints and helps to keep your heart and bones healthy. While walking at a slow pace (3.5 mph) for half an hour, a 155-pound person consumes 149 calories, raises the speed to 4 mph, and the same person burns 167calories.

Of course, running burns calories at the same time, but walking is an approachable, low-impact exercise that works for the majority. (Bonus points for exercising in nature: free-spending time has a lot of physical, social, and emotional benefits.) For regular weight loss, you'll need to watch at least twenty minutes of brisk walking most days of the week.

2. Lifting Weights:

It not only helps you burn fat, but also improves your ability to perform daily tasks such as carrying grocery stores, climbing stairs, and other household tasks. Lifting weights is critical because each year, we all lose one to two percent of our muscle strength. Free weight resistance training is crucial to weight loss; plus, right leg and hip muscles reduce your risk of falling, which is a significant cause of impairment in older adults.

Montoya recommends strength training at least twice a week for the lifting of newbies, with workouts being divided between upper-body exercises one day and lower-body exercises the other.

Tip: Skip the resistance machines and keep increasing your lifting weight as soon as it gets quick.

Older people tend to use only resistance machines, but I prefer using free weights because they require strength, and they enable more joint stabilizer muscle activity.

3. Yoga:

Not only does yoga make your muscles stronger, but it also increases your flexibility. Another advantage: during yoga, stretching and breathing deeply helps to reduce stress hormones that contribute to belly fat, a common problem for anyone over 50 years old. And since yoga lowers levels of stress, it also has the potential to improve your overall eating habits (less stress eating!), thus promoting weight loss.

Indeed, a study shows men lost fat by committing to a 14-week yoga program. The study people practiced 90 minutes of yoga five days a week, but don't worry, every little bit counts.

4. Interval Training:

If you're up for it, high-intensity interval training (HIIT), which is any workout where you alternate between intense activity and less intense activity, will help you burn more calories. It's one of the effective ways to lose weight, as long as you have permission from your doctor for strenuous exercise.

For older people, just starting out the best HIIT activities include swimming and cycling. You will see significant improvements in your aerobic fitness, strength, and blood-pressure readings by doing somewhat hard intervals, followed by easy intervals.

For the best results, Montoya suggests these intervals: five minutes of brisk walking, followed by five minutes of casual walking, three minutes on, three minutes rest, one-minute rest, one-minute rest and repeat. One can find the same pattern on the bike or in the pool. Start three days a week with a 30-minute workout period, and work up from there.

10.1 Build Lean Muscle Rapidly

Particularly in the weight room, patience is overrated, and especially when it comes to those concentrating on a particular outcome: muscle development.

Change takes time, of course, but if you're struggling to grow and build muscle, and don't see any noticeable increase in size from month to month, it's a sign your approach is off. And a workout is a dreadful thing to waste on. Plus, even if you see progress, there is no reason for you not to see more.

How do you revive your performance? There are nine ways here.

1. Increase Your Training Volume:

Training volume multiplied by your number of sets, your number of reps is a primary determinant of hypertrophy (aka how to grow muscle). And in order to increase volume, you might actually have to go down in weight than you might think.

Similar to strength training, the intensity will decrease during a program's hypertrophy process, with intensity sitting between 50 and 75 percent of the person's 1RM, the maximum weight he or she can lift for one rep. Do each of the lifts for three to six sets of 10 to 20 reps 2 to get the amount the muscles need.

2. Focus on the Eccentric Phase:

If you lift some weight, you have a concentrate (hard) and an eccentric phase (easy). For example, as you descend into a squat, you are performing a strange action. That is the focus when you return to standing. Yet the eccentric study is far stronger at causing hypertrophy, according to studies.

To maximize your workout's amount of eccentric effort, you can do two things: either slow down the strange process of each exercise you perform or incorporate unusual variations into your routine.

Take the squat, for example; you'd lower to the floor to make it eccentric-only, and end the exercise there. Note: If you're trying exercise-only, you'll need to increase the weight you're using substantially. Physiologically, muscles move eccentrically far stronger than they do concentrative.

3. Reduce Between-Set Rest Intervals:

If you are touching your phone between exercise sets, it is better to set the timer to 30 to 90 seconds. Rest periods of 30 to 90 seconds when lifting for hypertrophy encourage a rapid release into muscle-building hormones (including testosterone and human growth hormone) while also ensuring that you really, really tire your muscles.

Research published last year suggests that fatigue of your muscles is a prerequisite for hypertrophy, regardless of the rep and set scheme. Don't get scared of feeling the pain.

4. Eat More Protein:

Training breaks down your muscles to grow muscle. Protein builds them up again. And the harder you lift workouts, the more important it is to consider protein intake to solidify recovery from the muscle-building foods.

For optimum protein growth, weight lifters need to eat 0.25 to 0.30 grams of protein per kilogram of body weight per meal, according to research from the University of Sterling. This works out to 20 to 24 grams of protein at each meal for a 175-pound male. You will get this in three to four eggs, a cup of Greek yogurt, or a protein scoop powder.

5. Focus on Calorie Surpluses, Not Deficits:

This can be hard to get used to, especially for those who are used to calorie counting in hopes of weight loss. But to build muscle mass most effectively quickly (meaning weight gained, not lost), you need to consume more calories than you burn every day.

That's because when your body feels it's in a calorie deficit because you're eating fewer calories than you're burning every day, it slows down the urge of your body to build new muscle. After all, if your body thinks that food is in short supply, having sole won't be the prime concern.

Aim at eating around 250 to 500 extra calories per day. So ensure all weight gained comes from the muscle; it is advisable that the majority of those calories come from protein. In a study conducted by the Pennington Biomedical Research Center in 2014, people who ate a high-calorie protein-rich diet stored about 45 percent of those calories as muscle, while those who followed a low-protein diet with the same number of calories stored 95 percent as fat.

6. Snack on Casein Before Bed:

Long common among bodybuilders, casein protein gradually absorbs into the bloodstream, ensuring that it keeps the muscles filled with amino acids longer than other protein forms such as whey and plant proteins. In one study of Medicine and Science in Sports and Exercise, consuming casein protein immediately before bed boosted the circulating amino acid levels of young men for 7.5 hours; they built muscle throughout the night while they were sleeping.

Try cottage cheese, Greek yogurt, and milk, to get some pre-bed casein. The casein-based protein powder works like a charm for smoothie lovers.

7. Get More Sleep:

 One needs more than the right nutrition to recover the muscle. Recovery time takes about eight hours per night. After all, the body releases human growth hormone as you sleep, which helps the tissue development and keeps the stress hormone cortisol levels in check.

Furthermore, a study shows that sleeping for five hours, as opposed to eight hours, reduces muscle-building testosterone levels by a whopping 10 to 15 percent every night for just one week.

The National Sleep Foundation suggests adults aged between 18 and 64 sleep seven to nine hours a night. No apologies.

8. Try to Add Creatine:

Creatine doesn't develop muscle directly. But the natural compound effectively promotes muscle growth by boosting your performance at high-intensity lifting workouts, according to study.

In fact, researchers concluded in one research review that creatine supplementation at a given weight could help you lift 14 percent more reps than you can without supplements.

Aim for creatine monohydrate; the supplement's most thoroughly researched type for best results.

9. HMB:

A natural compound, beta-hydroxyl-beta-methyl butyrate, developed in the human body, prevents muscle-protein breakdown, promotes muscle growth, and accelerates exercise recovery.

Unfortunately, through food alone, it is hard to increase the levels significantly. It is here that supplementation comes in. For example, taking HMB in tandem with a high-intensity lifting regimen significantly improved muscle strength and size relative to lifting alone, in a 12-week resistance-trained individual study. Besides, HMB helps prevent the consequences of overtraining like loss of muscle in the off-chance that you are working yourself too hard.

Chapter 11: Recipes that Help in Intermittent Fasting

Don't know what to eat at irregular fasts? Get the most out of your weight-loss journey with science-backed ultimate intermittent fasting food list.

It can be confusing to eat during intermittent fasting (IF). This is because IF is not a diet plan but rather a pattern of eating. Keeping this in mind, Do Fasting experts have developed an intermittent list of fasting foods that will keep you healthy while you're on your weight loss journey.

IF tells you when to eat but doesn't mention what foods your diet can include. A lack of clear dietary guidelines can give a misleading impression that you can eat anything you want. For others, choosing the "right" foods and drinks will cause problems.

11.1 Breakfast:

Here, we describe the few foods you can use in your breakfast while doing the intermittent fasting.

1. Egg White Omelette with Cherry Tomatoes

Egg whites are a good choice if you cut back on calories because the egg white contains just 18 calories.

SERVES 1PREP 5 Minutes COOK for 5 Minutes

- 3 Large Eggs (54 Cal's For Egg Whites)

- 1 Tbsp. Skimmed Milk (5 Cal's)

- 3 Light Sunflower Oil Sprays (3 Cal's)

- 10 Cherry Tomatoes, Cut In Half (22 Cal's)

- Fresh basil leaves, broken (optional) salt and freshly ground black pepper

- Separate the eggs first. Crack one of the eggs on a clean bowl's edge, and open the two halves using your thumbs, letting some of the white spills into the bowl.

- Move the egg yolk cautiously, making the egg white spill into the cup, from one half of the shell to another.

- Keep passing the yolk of the egg from one half of the tank to the other without breaking it until the bowl is entirely white. Place the yolk in a separate bowl and reuse the remaining 2 eggs.

- Add the milk to the whites of the egg, and whisk with a fork.

- Sprinkle the oil in a large frying pan (skillet) and cook for at least 2 minutes over medium heat; Pour the white mixture into the bowl, then quickly add the cherry tomatoes and basil.

- Season with salt and pepper and continue cooking until finished.

- You may need to swirl and tilt the pan uniformly over the base of the pan to spread the eggs, tomatoes, and basil.

- The omelet will cook in under a minute.

- Directly serve.

2. Spinach and Mushroom Egg White Frittata

For a quick and balanced breakfast, fresh spinach and sliced mushrooms are sautéed and cooked with egg whites, then topped with salty parmesan cheese.

Just a few ingredients are needed to make this egg white frittata super healthy and comfortable with spinach, mushrooms, and parmesan!

Preparation Time is 5 minutes, Cook Time 10 minutes and Total Time 15 minutes

Ingredients:

- 2-3 sliced brown mushrooms

- A handful of fresh spinach

- 1 cup of white egg

- Kosher salt

- 2 tablespoons grated Parmesan cheese

- Hot sauce if needed

Procedure:

- Preheat the oven to broil, or toaster.

- Sprinkle a7-inch non-stick fry pan with medium-heat cooking spray and hot. Attach the sliced mushrooms and cook, turning once or twice, for 2-3 minutes. Attach the spinach fresh and cook for 1-2 minutes or until the spinach wilts.

- In a cup, whisk the egg whites until light and shiny, add a pinch of kosher salt and dump into the mushroom and spinach mix.

- Add 1 tablespoon of parmesan to sprinkle.

- Let the eggs cook untouched until the edges of the egg whites begin to cook through, making a more solid white. Lift the sides of the egg whites gently and raise the saucepan so that the uncooked egg runs under the cooked portion and cook for another minute.

- Switch the frying pan to the oven and broil for 2-3 minutes, or until the eggs have puffed through and fried.

- Remove from the frying pan and sprinkle with the remaining parmesan cheese.

- Cut into wedges, and serve as needed with hot sauce.

3. Carrot Salad

Salad is a healthy breakfast for you, and it also helps you to maintain your intermittent fasting. Here is the simple recipe for making carrot salad for breakfast.

Eight ingredients are needed:

- 2 Beets, large

- 2 Carrots, medium

- 2 Granny smith apples

- 1/4 cup 2 lemons, Zest & Juice

- 1/2 tbsp. Honey, raw Baking & Spices

- 1/2 tbsp. Black pepper

- 3/4 tbsp. Sea salt Oils & Vinegar

- 1 tbsp. Olive oil

The Procedure of Making:

- Shred the beets, carrots, and apples. You can choose to use a food processor or a box grater. Place the shredded beets, carrots, and apples into a big bowl.
- Zest the lemons, and add it to the bowl. Cut the lemons and squeeze out the juice into the bowl.
- Add the olive oil, salt, pepper, and honey to taste.
- Toss the salad well in order to combine evenly all the ingredients.
- Keeps in the fridge for up to 2-3 days.

4. Garlic Butter Sauteed Zucchini

Seasoned Zucchini is a quick, easy, and healthy side dish. It's yummy too. I love this version with garlic and butter cooked met Zucchini. You only need to prepare for five minutes, and it is time to eat! Jump to the Sautéed Zucchini Garlic Butter Recipe or read on to see our tips for making it.

How to Cook Zucchini on Stove:

There are plenty of ways to cook Zucchini, but pan-frying or sautéing it in a pot on the stove is the quickest way. In this way, by cooking Zucchini, the Zucchini browns outwardly and becomes soft internally.

- When the Zucchini is fried in a small butter, pan-fry it. The butter adds a nutty flavor and helps brown the Zucchini.

- Add a spoonful of hazelnut garlic to the plate because butter and garlic are meant to be, right? The secret to sauté the Zucchini isn't overcooking it. Overcooked courgettes grow mushy.

Potential Zucchini Recipe Variations:

Sautéed Zucchini has many possible variations in the recipes. Here are some of the favorites:

- Make it cheesy, and just before serving, stir in some grated parmesan or some other type of cheese.

- We love garlic and butter blends, but you can use other spices. Try Italian seasoning, Za'atar spice mix, Cajun seasoning, an Indian spice blend such as curry powder, or chili powder (here's our homemade powder blend).

- Add the toasted sliced almonds or buttery pine nuts in some extra crunch.

- Drop the Zucchini in chopped tomatoes and cook until the Zucchini is crisp and the tomatoes crumble a little, releasing some of their juices.

- By adding cooked or canned beans, add more protein — white beans, chickpeas, and black beans would be excellent.

11.2 Lunch:

1. Turmeric Rack of Lamb

It is such an easy-breezy recipe, but the end result is so tender and juicy. The turmeric and garlic add to this dish such a great flavor, and along with the lemon, they are a delicious combo.

Ingredients:

- 1.5 lb. of lamb rib chops

- 1 tbsp. of extra virgin olive oil

- 1 tbsps. of lemon juice

- One lemon zest

- Four minced garlic cloves

- 1 1/2 tbsp. of salt

- 1/2 tbsp. of turmeric powder

- 1/2 tbsp. of dried oregano

- 1 tbsp. of coconut oil

Instructions:

- Pat dry the lamb with a paper towel, then use a sharp knife to slice between each rib to separate the chops two if they are not already separated. To form a paste mix, extra virgin olive oil, lemon juice, lemon zest, garlic, sea salt, turmeric powder, and dried oregano.

- Rub this lamb paste marinade all over. Cover-marinate in the fridge for a total of 30 minutes to 1 hour.

- Heat the coconut oil over medium heat in a large skillet.

- Take the lamb from the fridge, and fry the lamb on each side for 3-4 minutes for medium-rare.

- Serve with your favorite.

2. BBQ Pork Tender

BBQ Pork Tenderloin made from marinade with a slice of sweet, zesty pork. For both grilled pork tenderloin and baked, this recipe is delicious! Always a favorite of the crowd!

Ingredients:

- 1 3-4 pound pork tenderloin

- 1/2 cup BBQ sauce

- 1/4 cup grape jelly

- Two tablespoons Sriracha sauce

- Two tablespoons Worcestershire amino sauce or coconut

- One clove minced garlic

- One tablespoon of ground black pepper black pepper

Instructions:

- Place the pork tenderloin in a large zip-top bag.

- Whisk the BBQ sauce, grape jelly, Sriracha sauce, Worcestershire sauce, garlic, and pepper together. Pour half a mixture of the BBQ sauce over the pork tenderloin. Remove excess air and seal from the zip-top bag. Put pork tenderloins in the fridge for an hour to marinate overnight. Cover leftover marinade/sauce with plastic wrap and place for later use in the refrigerator.

- Bake 425 degrees F. And barbecue pork tenderloins until they exceed 160 degrees F indoors. Clear from the oven or grill and place for 5 to 10 minutes to rest in covered glass or ceramic casserole dish.

Brush with an extra BBQ sauce when ready to serve. Serve with additional side sauce.

3. Fish Bars:

The ingredients for the fish bars are absolutely fuss-free and can probably be found right this minute in your pantry.

Ingredients:

- Vegetable oil for frying

- 1/3 cup all-purpose flour

- Two large eggs

- 1/2 teaspoon baking powder

- 1/2 teaspoon salt

- 1/2 cup beer or milk

- Salt and pepper

- 1 pound of haddock or cod fillets cut into strips

Instructions:

- Heat oil over medium, high heat in a medium-sized bowl.

- In a medium-sized bowl, whisk together the flour, eggs, baking powder, and salt until smooth.

- Next, mix gradually in beer or milk and whisk until batter is mixed.

- Then dip each piece into batter coating evenly with salt and pepper.

- In grease, fry the fish until golden brown and crispy.

- Next, fry until golden brown.

- Season with salt and pepper and drink.

4. Artichoke Petals Bites

Ingredients:

- 1 cup (50 g) panko bread crumbs

- 1/2 cup (60 g) vegetarian parmesan cheese

- 1/2 cup (125 mL) salted butter, one-piece, melted

- 15 oz. (425 g) canned artichoke core, two cans, drained, rinsed, and patted dry fresh parsley, minced, to be eaten.

Garlic Aioli:

- 1/2 cup (115 g) mayonnaise

- Two tablespoons of olive oil

- One teaspoon of garlic, hazelnut

- One tablespoon of lemon juice

- 1/4 teaspoon of salt

- 1/4 cup (10 g) of new, chopped parsley;

Preparation:

- Preheat the oven until 200oC (400 ° F). Line a parchment-paper baking sheet and inside placed a wire rack.

- Drain the artichokes and rinse. Press them over warm.

- Combine the brown crumbs and vegetarian Parmesan cheese in a medium bowl.

- In the melted butter, dip the artichoke hearts to ensure they are adequately coated. Then cover well with a mixture of bread crumbs.

- Place the bites of the artichoke onto the rack.

- Bake for 15 minutes, then reduce the temperature of the oven to 350oF (175oC), flip the artichokes, and bake for another 15 minutes until the heart of the artichokes is warmed and the mixture of bread crumbs is toasted.

- While doing so, make the garlic aioli. Combine the mayonnaise, olive oil, garlic, lemon juice, butter, and parsley in a small bowl. Stir to merge.

- Sprinkle with parsley on the artichoke bites before serving alongside with aioli.

- Love it!

11.3 Snacks:

1. Butternut Squash Bites

Just seven ingredients are needed to make this festive appetizer, and most of the parts are probably already in your pocket!

Ingredients:

- One box of 15 shells of frozen mini phyllo dough

- 1, 10 oz. Frozen butternut squash bag

- 1 Tbsp. Unsalted butter

- 1/4 medium white onion, finely diced

- 1/4 cup thin, shredded cheddar cheese

- 2 tbsp. Clean basil, chopped to taste

- Salt and pepper

- 1/4 tbsp. Red chili flakes

- Garnish with pumpkin seeds

Instructions:

- Heat oven to 375 ° F. Place the shells on a baking sheet. Then, frozen butternut squash microwave as indicated on the box.

- Melt butter and cook onion in a medium-sized skillet over medium heat for ~5 minutes, occasionally stirring. The onion will become almost translucent.

- Mash the butternut squash in a medium bowl, using a potato masher.

- Stir in the cooked onions, cheese, sage, and seasonings until they are beautifully incorporated.

- Mix phyllo shells in a spoon and bake for 8 minutes. Fill with ground seeds and serve warm.

2. Pepperoni Pizza Bites:

Pepperoni Bites are a cross between a muffin pizza and a bagel slice and are ready to bake in just a few minutes.

Ingredients:

- 3/4 cup meal

- 3/4 teaspoon baking powder

- 3/4 cup 2% milk

- 1 egg, slightly beaten

- 1 teaspoon Italian seasoning

- 1/4 teaspoon crushed red pepper

- 1/4 teaspoon salt

- 1/2 cup mozzarella cheese

- 1/2 cup Parmesan cheese

- 4.2 ounces pepperoni (Half the bag, cut into small quarters)

Instructions:

- Oven preheats to 375 ° C. For one pan, add the milk and eggs, set aside.

- Mix the flour, baking powder, salt, Italian seasoning, and crushed red pepper in a second bowl.

- Mix the wet into the dry ingredients and mix with a whisk.

- Put the pepperoni and cheese together and whisk in.

- Spray the baking spray or spray the canola oil onto two mini muffin tins and fill all 24 with 1 tablespoon scoop.

- Alternatively, make the Pepperoni Pizza Bites 12 bigger.

- Cook for 15-18 minutes, or until golden.

- Serve with Marinara Mezzetta Sauce

3. Chicken Strips:

Ingredients:

- 2-2/3 cups of salt (about 80 crackers)

- 1 teaspoon of garlic salt

- 1/2 teaspoon of dried basil

- 1/2 teaspoon of paprika

- 1/8 teaspoon of pepper

- 1 large egg

- 1 cup of whole milk

- 1-1/2 pound of boneless skinless chicken breasts, sliced into 1/2-inch pieces

- Frying oil

Preparation:

- Combine the first 5 ingredients into a shallow bowl. Place the egg and milk in yet another shallow dish. Dip the chicken into a mixture of the eggs, then cover it with the cracker.

- Heat oil to 375 ° C in an electric skillet or deep-fat fryer. Fry the chicken, a couple of stripes at a time, on each side for 2-3 minutes, or until golden brown. Drain on towels made from paper.

11.4 Dinner:

It leads to a complete 24-hour fast by fasting from dinner one day to dinner the next. It's essential after 24 hours fasting that you can take a healthy diet.

1. Curried Rice

For a tremendous Curried Rice, you need more than just curry powder!! Basmati gives a perfectly nutty flavor to this rice recipe. Spiciness: Dry, not overly spicy. Not supposed to be a full-on authentic Indian recipe, but it leans more to Indian than flavorful Western curry recipes.

Ingredients

- 3 tbsp. of yellow curry powder

- 1 tbsp. of cumin

- 1 tbsp. of coriander

- 1/2 tbsp. of paprika

- 1/2 tbsp. of chili powder

RICE:

- 40 g/3 tbsp. butter (or ghee or oil) 1 onion, finely chopped

- 3 garlic cloves, minced

- 2 tbsp. of ginger, finely chopped or rubbed

- 1 1/2 cups of basmati rice, uncooked

- 2 small carrots, peeled and rubbed

- 2 1/4 cups of chicken or vegetable broth, low sodium

- 2 cups of frozen peas

- 1 1/4 tbsp. of salt

- 1/2 tbsp. of black pepper

- 1 cup (150 g) cashews, roasted, unsalted

- 1/2 cup coriander/cilantro leaves, finely chopped

- Yogurt (optional) for serving.

Directions:

- Rinse rice until it runs relatively clear, and drain well.

- Melt butter over medium, high heat in a small to medium pot (or large saucepan).

- Attach ginger and garlic, and cook for 30 seconds. Add the onion and cook until slightly translucent, for 2 minutes.

- Add carrot and cook, until soft and sweet, for 2-3 minutes.

- Add rice and whisk in the oil to coat all the seeds.

- Add spices to cover the rice and blend.

- Remove broth, peas, pepper, and salt, and mix. If any rice protrudes above the surface, poke it beneath the liquid.

- When the entire surface of the liquid is simmering, swirl once, put the lid on and turn the heat down to LOW immediately.

- Cook 14 minutes, don't peek while you cook!

- Lift lid slightly and quickly tilts pot to test for the absorption of liquid. Clamp the lid back on and take-off power.

- Live undisturbed for 10 minutes.

- Use a rubber spatula to flake rice gently.

- Add most of the cashews and cilantro, and mix.

- Transfer to bowl serving, sprinkle with remaining cashews and cilantro. See in post for suggestions to represent.

2. Pan-Fried Cod:

Ingredients:

In The Coleslaw:

- 1/2 cup mayonnaise

- 2 tablespoons of apple cider vinegar

- 1 tablespoon of whole-grain mustard and more to eat

- 1 tablespoon of sugar

- 1/4 to 1/2 teaspoon of caraway or celery seeds

- Cowshed salt and freshly ground pepper

- 1/2 head of light green cabbage, thinly sliced (about 6 cups)

- 1 small carrot, shredded

- 1 gala apple, julienned

- 1 bunch of scallions, white a bunch of scallions

Directions

- Prepare the slaw: mix in a large bowl with the mayonnaise, vinegar, mustard, sugar, caraway seeds, 1 1/2 teaspoon salt, and pepper to taste. Toss the cabbage, the carrot, the apple, and the scallions; cover and cool off.

- Prepare the fish: In a medium bowl, whisk the egg and milk; add the cod and set aside for soaking. Mix on a platter the rice, the cracker meal, the cayenne pepper, and a pinch of salt.

- Remove the fish from the mixture of milk, and dredge in the mix of flour, turning to coat. Fry in the hot oil for 2 to 4 minutes per side until golden.

- Transfer to a drain plate lined with paper towels; season with salt and pepper.

- Serve with the mustard and extra slaw.

Conclusion

When making dietary changes, it is always best to consult with a trained healthcare professional, even if you just change the timing when you eat food. They can help you figure out if intermittent fasting would be right for you. This is particularly important for long-term fasts where there may be vitamin and mineral depletion. It's essential to understand how incredibly smart our bodies are. The body will increase appetite and the number of calories consumed at the next meal if food is limited at one meal, and even slow down the metabolism to match calorie consumption.

Intermittent fasting has many potential health benefits, but it should not be assumed that, if strictly followed, massive weight loss is guaranteed, and disease development or progression prevented. It is a useful tool, but it may need to implement many tools to help.

References

Healthline. (n.d.). What Is Intermittent Fasting? Explained in Human Terms. [online] Available at: https://www.healthline.com/nutrition/what-is-intermittent-fasting.

Dr. Jason Fung, M. (n.d.). The 7 practical benefits of fasting - Diet Doctor. [online] Diet Doctor. Available at: https://www.dietdoctor.com/7-benefits-of-fasting.

Healthline. (n.d.). 11 Ways to Boost Human Growth Hormone (HGH) Naturally. [online] Available at: https://www.healthline.com/nutrition/11-ways-to-increase-hgh#1.

Healthline. (n.d.). 6 Popular Ways to Do Intermittent Fasting. [online] Available at: https://www.healthline.com/nutrition/6-ways-to-do-intermittent-fasting#section7.

Publishing, H. (n.d.). 9 tips to boost your energy — naturally - Harvard Health. [online] Harvard Health. Available at: https://www.health.harvard.edu/energy-and-fatigue/9-tips-to-boost-your-energy-naturally.

LIFE Apps | LIVE and LEARN. (n.d.). The 5 Stages of Intermittent Fasting - LIFE Apps | LIVE and LEARN. [online] Available at: https://lifeapps.io/fasting/the-5-stages-of-intermittent-fasting/.

Dr Becky Fitness. (n.d.). Intermittent Fasting for Women Over 50 - Good or Bad?. [online] Available at: https://www.drbeckyfitness.com/intermittent-fasting-for-women-over-50/.

James Clear. (n.d.). The Beginner's Guide to Intermittent Fasting. [online] Available at: https://jamesclear.com/the-beginners-guide-to-intermittent-fasting.

K. Aleisha Fetters, C., K. Aleisha Fetters, C., Editors, T., Editors, T., Editors, T. and Editors, T. (n.d.). Grow Muscle: 9 Proven Ways to Build Muscle Fast | Spartan Race. [online] Spartan Life. Available at: https://life.spartan.com/post/grow-muscle.